THE NEW REALITY OF NUTRIENTS

Making Sense of Vitamins, Minerals, Supplements, and Herbs

Dr. David L. Vastola, D. O

W & B Publishers
USA

W & B Publishers

For information:
W & B Publishers
9001 Ridge Hill Street
Kernersville, NC 27284

www.a-argusbooks.com

ISBN: 9781635540994

Book Cover designed by Dubya

Printed in the United States of America

Dedication

I dedicate this book to my best friend, my lifetime
companion, my wife Gail.
She has always been there for me.

To my medical school and medical residency/fellowship
programs that taught and made me what I am today.

Disclaimer: This book should only be used as a reference and only used in the context of standard medical care with your physician. Your doctor is ultimately responsible for your care, and any uses other than those described above would be considered ill advised. Also, the interrelationship between vitamins, minerals, supplements, herbs, and other medications should be evaluated by your doctor.

CONTENTS

Introduction

Constant research and new revelations in the field of nutritional supplements and their benefits have created a frequently changing landscape. One recent example (and there are countless others), found antioxidants have helped some veterans with PTSD (Post Traumatic Stress Disorder). But even with outstanding evidence, the prudent consumer should not randomly buy all the nutritional supplements advertised. Supplements must be used with professional medical supervision by someone who has had the applicable education and training. Knowing how nutrient therapies work will add to their usefulness, which is why I'm thrilled with the world-class research being done. Ignorance is bliss, but not when it comes to living a longer and happier life.

As a basic strategy, everyone needs a complete physical every year, with a full range of tests recommended by your physician. The nutrients can then be tailored to the patient's needs and diagnosed in accordance to the results of these tests.

As sad as it sounds, the human body deteriorates daily; sometimes able to heal and regenerate itself if properly cared for by what we subject it to environmentally (the quality of air and water), nutritionally (what we eat, drink, and otherwise consume), what we allow on our skin (the largest organ and least cared for; over-exposure to the sun, lotions, detergents, hygiene products, cleaning chemicals, etc.), and what we listen to, watch, and subject ourselves to (radio, TV, internet —

emotionally, physically, and socially). If you abuse it, you lose it. We can't always control certain variables, but most we can... should we choose to. As in the Garden of Eden, we have decisions to make every second of every day. Those choices determine our mental, physical, and spiritual health.

Your body, if not abused, has all it needs to keep going as long as some disease does not come along and "take you out." A complete physical every year with a competent doctor, who takes a genuine interest in your well-being, is the key. Any illness could end your search for optimal health. You must have the mindset: Prevention is much better than treatment.

As ridiculous as it sounds, new patients have come into my office with two and three trays of the vitamins; wasting hundreds of dollars every month and for no good reason. Purchasing and consuming them may make people feel good psychologically (via the placebo effect), but medically, at best, doing so is only marginally helpful and may even be harmful. Taking supplements without medical advice can deprive people of proper medical care.

To understand the concept of aging, to find the elusive answers, we need to not only go back to review and consider ancient findings and studies, but also seek out the truth behind what we are bombarded with daily on TV, radio, the internet, in publications, and in doctors' offices concerning healthcare, pharmaceuticals, nutrients, supplements, skin care products, etc. The list is as long as infinity. Yet, the truth will not be found in disclaimers, in the examples of celebrities, or a guru's pouch but rather within yourself. And to open its secret, you must understand the four mechanisms or vehicles that'll get you there.

Perhaps the most important mechanism to longevity goes back to genetics and DNA. Within this genetic category, I have identified three subcategories which, in turn leads:

1. Your inherited genetics.
2. Telomeres.
3. Mitochondria.

Genetics

Your genetics are mirrored through your family history, and are important to your doctor. They give clues to what may be affecting you and what the future may hold. You know the old expression 'the past repeats itself'? Well, that can happen to you through your own genetics. For example, if you have a family history of heart disease or breast or prostate cancer, then your chances are higher of experiencing these life-threatening problems. It is not guaranteed, but it all should be taken into serious consideration. Be very suspicious of doctors who do not take a good family history; this is a significant oversight.

Telomeres

The second subcategory is telomeres, the end amino-acid sequences of our DNA molecules. As we get older, they start to shorten. With this shortening, the cell can no longer reproduce itself in a timely manner, thus decreasing its life span, which in turn leads to organ dysfunction. External factors, such as smoking, excessive alcohol use, and free radicals from oxidation, hurt them.

Free radicals are molecules that have lost an outer ring electron, making them very active and angry. They adversely affect cells with inflammation and, over time, are associated with DNA mutations and cancer.

Another is EMFs (electromagnetic fields) from all the electronic devices surrounding us — cell phones, computers, routers, etc. — are forms of radiation that destroy the DNA. After the bombs at Hiroshima and Nagasaki, cancer was a big problem for this very reason. Sometimes many overlapping fields exist, like concentric rings, called EMF Fog. Here are some of the more important references:

1. Electro smog — the summation of all the EMFs in an environment.
2. HFVT (High-frequency voltage transits) — power companies now emit a pulsed electrical current to our neighborhoods to save energy. But in doing so, these create a back and forth EMF that never leaves our homes and work places, accumulating effects on our DNA.
3. Hypersensitivity — some people are allergic to these EMFs and, as a result, have vague symptoms of headache, fatigue, tinnitus, low-grade temperature, muscle aches, and pains. Sound familiar? Fibromyalgia or chronic fatigue syndrome? These new technological advances have created a whole new genre of human diseases, including a loss of our telomeres.

Mitochondria

The third part of the genetic cause for aging is our cellular mitochondria. Many experts, such as Dr. Bruce Aims at the University of California, have postulated for years that aging was a function of losing our mitochondria. I agree completely. Mitochondria are the energy-making part of our cells, like the gas tanks of our cars, which have their own DNA separate from the nuclear DNA. The new science says longevity directly parallels them.

Normally, we have 2-2000 mitochondria per cell. But as we age, the mitochondria decrease in number, leading to a loss of intracellular energy, causing organ dysfunction and aging. Researchers have identified acetyl-L-carnitine, branched chain amino acids, CoQ10, and lipoic acid as ways of not only maintaining these mitochondria but also increasing their numbers (biogenesis). Regardless, mitochondria are important players and we need to consider them as they pertain to aging.

Hormone and Enzyme Deficiency:

The fourth and last of the mechanisms for optimal health is the raw materials necessary for our metabolic engines, the very essence of this book. Our diet, or any diet for that matter, cannot supply these materials in adequate amounts. Therefore, without a doubt, supplements are necessary. DHAE (dihydroepiandrosterone) was the first hormone linked to aging and age-related in decreased amounts. A Dr. Vladimer Dilman in his 1960 paper "Health Project," reported this very thing. Now we know that many other hormones and needed enzymes do the same thing.

As a corollary, I have adopted the term, "antioxidant bank," which is a buildup of antioxidants to neutralize any free radicals floating around. In doing so, you can pre-empt any damage resulting from free radicals before symptoms occur. They do it by donating an electron from their outer ring, which the free radicles need and will then decrease their reactivity.

I must remind you, supplementation needs to accompany exercise; nutrients alone will not work. Just like your car, you can have all the gasoline you need, but without maintenance, the engine will stop running and your journey through life will end abruptly. It amazes and astounds me to this day how people take better care of their cars and boats than their own bodies.

Incidentally, these "meat markets," what we call our exercise facilities, may help with our health requirements in a small way, and *only* small. This mostly encourages a "body yard sale." Don't delude yourself into thinking that having a great-looking body or six-pack correlates to great or even good health. Your inner appearance is what counts, not the external one. We will discuss in detail about what exercise is all about later.

My guess is that once you have read this book, several things will happen. First, you will start thinking as a medical profession would; researching and understanding more about your body and environment. Next, you will be able to ask relevant questions and intelligently seek out what you need. This is really a reorientation, a quest that will draw everything together, like a sneaker with loose shoe strings calling out to be tightened up. Yes, the didactics help, but the overview is even more important, as then it becomes your game plan.

As a university professor, my main objective is to make my students think. I use the Socratic Method; asking questions of my students, hoping it prompts them to rationalize the answers. Otherwise, you will only retain 20% of what you read or are taught. This book is my attempt to make you think and say, "Wow, that makes sense!" You will see knowing and using the facts is the magic formula for optimal health.

Last, don't be afraid to ask your doctor *any* question, and *don't* base your decisions purely on what you find on the Internet or your neighbor when it comes to medical advice. Do your research, take notes, make an appointment with your doctor, and seek out a new one if yours will not listen or is not open to alternative medicine. It is essential to have a physician who is interested in integrating all forms of medicine — Eastern Western, Holistic, Traditional, Alternative, Chiropractic, etc. The answer to your health issue may not be found in just one but a little of everything! It's amazing how many so-called experts are out there with no medical education to legitimatize their information. These 'experts' could exacerbate your problems, cause others to form, or actually be responsible for ending your life should you take something that contraindicates with what you are taking now, triggers an allergic reaction, or even shuts down organs. Supplements can affect everything. Be sure before you pop a pill. For me, I am constantly studying and learning, and I practice what I teach.

On a recent trip, my wife ran out of suitcase space and asked if I had room in my bag to take some of her things.

I said, "Of course."

After a short time struggling with the room available, she shouted, "Do you know how many vitamin bottles — more accurately, nutritional bottles — you have in this suitcase? Nineteen!"

And because of them, she could not get her stuff in.

I responded, "I take more daily. That's why I'm seventy years of age going on fifty, or maybe forty."

She smirked.

This is not meant to be a self-validation for what I do, but instead an example for you. This book's content has proven research and will help you succeed with your own quest for health!

Chapter One

How Things Work

A good way to start this journey is to approach the most commonly asked questions, and in so doing, eliminate much of the lingering doubts and misconceptions you may have.

We all share the quest for longevity. And, as mentioned earlier, supplying and maintaining your metabolic engines is the main thrust of *The New Reality of Nutrients*. Nutrition in partnership with exercise is powerful. I recommend using the knowledge within these pages as your yardstick. Even college nutrition courses lack insight into modern research on nutritional therapies and dosages. For example, the RDAs (recommended daily allowances) are foolishly outdated, i.e., vitamin C with an RDA of 70 mg/day, when, in fact, the most effective dose is 2000 for women/3000 for men mg/day!

Credentials

A short review of my background will help you understand my intimate relationship with nutrient therapies. My medical training is a bit hybrid. I graduated from an osteopathic medical school in Chicago (Midwestern University) with honors, but finished my internal medicine residency and gastroenterology fellowship at MD institutions, obtaining my MD certifications in both.

I was then accepted at the Mayo Clinic for a research fellowship in gastroenterology immunology, but at the last minute decided to stay at the University of Buffalo as chief of gastroenterology at the Deaconess Hospital. I taught there for five years in the schools of medicine and pharmacy, and at Buffalo's Children's Hospital, obtaining a position on the prestigious medical school admissions committee, which I truly loved. I then left for private practice in Florida, where I am today, taking care of patients with internal medicine or gastroenterology problems. I also continue to teach nutrition at the School of Pharmacy at Palm Beach Atlantic University, where I have been for ten years.

For twenty years, I had a live radio show in southern Florida. I also contributed to the local Fox TV station 10 o'clock news for eight years, five nights weekly, where I frequently discussed medical and nutritional issues.

Now you might ask, where did he get his education and information regarding nutritional therapies? I am self-taught. I had a genuine interest in it for my patients, and it was mandatory for the live radio program. Since the 80s, more people have become health conscious, and with the listener's nutritional questions, I had better know the answers.

Over the decades, I've honed my nutritional therapies; not only vitamins, minerals, and trace elements, but also herbal remedies, and Ayurvedic ones from India. And yes, eating Indian food, such as curry, will help. These Indian remedies consist of two groups, Rasa and Shastra. Shastra use with caution because many contain heavy metals that should be explicitly avoided, and the ones sold on the Internet are especially dangerous.

Nutritional therapies are far from new. The history of nutritional supplements goes all the way back to the ancient Egyptian Imhotep, who lived around the 27th Century BC, and is considered by many to be the true father of medicine. His honey remedy for skin infections is still as effective as the standard topical antibiotics we use today. So, if you are on a picnic and someone gets a cut or scratch, reach for the raw honey!

The next pivotal medical figure in the time line is Hippocrates, the ancient Greek who lived around 460 BC, and is also considered the father of medicine. His writings of medical and surgical therapies are considered very sophisticated for his time.

More recently, Dr. Linus Pauling, a two-time Noble Prize winner in chemistry, advocated the use of extremely high doses of vitamin C to fight infections, and Dr. Paul Brunwald at Harvard believed in fish oils (omega-3 EPA) to prevent disease.

Finally, and with all humility, for thirty years on radio, television, and with my own patients, I have promoted the idea of nutritional supplements, along with the standard medical conventional treatments.

People encounter many problems when it comes to sorting out nutritional therapies. Perhaps the worst is the Internet, which is full of incorrect and useless information, all done to make a quick buck. The "pollution highway," I call it, should be avoided at all costs. More problematic are the self-proclaimed experts. They know everything from brain surgery to hangnails, and yet most do not have one speck of medical training or experience.

Perhaps more insidious is the problem of inconsistencies. The University of Alabama School of Pharmacy did an interesting study years ago where they sent students into the same nutritional stores or pharmacies to ask the same questions over a certain time. They found the recommendations were *never* the same. And the reason: no one knew the correct answer, including the clerks, pharmacists, and doctors alike.

Mechanisms of Action

Understanding physiology (how things work) and nomenclature (the medical language) will help you understand how to use nutritional therapies. Now, let's take a closer look.

Human cell reproduction, no matter where it is — liver, kidneys, heart, gall bladder — requires raw materials for its metabolic engines without interference. Interference can be caused by toxic materials, loss of blood supply, alcohol, smoking, and free radicals (electron-seeking molecules) that disrupt the cellular reproductive process. If left intact (without interference), organs, such as your liver and kidneys, will replace themselves every seven years; your heart, every twenty-eight years. Forever. This is why you see some people in 3rd-world countries live to be 120 years old. Their food, water, and air have not been contaminated, and they walk just about everywhere they go — exercise. This is fundamental to understanding these therapies over a long time — not a week or a month or two. I have outlined these mechanisms and will now explain.

Immunity

Our immunity is our first-line defense against bacteria, viruses, and fungal infections. During the first six months of life, you share your mother's immunity until your own kicks in. Breastfeeding for longer periods extends this — two-plus years or longer is optimal — and waiting to introduce solids ensures a healthier GI track, and as everyone knows, it all refers back to the digestive track. Breastmilk is the superior infant food. La Leche League has been promoting this for nearly seventy years. But it actually starts with the mother's health even before conception — genetics, inherited issues, diet, environment, exercise, habits. Without an effective immune system, we would eventually die from infection, and yes, cancer, too, since this same system kills tumor cells before they have a chance to grow.

Now let me review for you how our immune system works.

Anything "foreign" needs to be processed first, and the immune system does this through specific cells (the sentries) called dendritics or macrophages. They engulf the invader, break it down, and then call in the specific cells to get rid of it. There are two lines of cells:

1. The "B" cells that attack bacteria through antibodies they produce.
2. "T" cells that kill fungus, viruses, and tumor cells. Chemicals called cytokines are initially helpful and drive the inflammation process. But if chronically in use, they lead to other problems, such as scarring with organ dysfunction and cancer.

Allergies are also part of this system, whether from hay fever, asthma, or bee stings, and operate the same way but through a "B" cell antibody (IgE). In a class of diseases called "autoimmune," the body reacts to its own cells, but we are not quite sure why. A few examples are lupus, sarcoid, Sjogren's, and scleroderma disease.

Immunosenescense, a more recent concept, describes why we are seeing shingles, mumps, and more cancer in older people because these mechanisms don't work as well. They simply "run out of immune gas." The fatigue in our immune systems sets us up for these problems. Hence, we are now recommending older people be vaccinated to ramp-up their immune-decrepit systems.

Since about twenty million people have exaggerated immune systems, manifesting as autoimmune diseases, an agent to suppress it safely would be ideal. It turns out peony and mung-bean extracts rebalance these reactions to re-establish homeostasis to a normal setting. The mechanism here includes a reduction of the inflammatory chemicals, which break the chains of inflammation. It also reduces tissue stimulation and overgrowth, along with slowing the maturation of cells promoting inflammation, and subsequently boosts the maturation of regulatory cells. Much like fish oils, it has a "stop-like" effect (putting on the brakes) to turn off the inflammatory reaction, which, in the case of autoimmune diseases, is out of control.

As mentioned earlier, lupus, Sjogren's syndrome, sarcoidosis, and scleroderma are some examples that can be vastly improved with peony and mung-bean extracts, along with lesser diseases, such as psoriasis, alopecia areata (localized bald spots), and iritis (inflammation of the outer part of the eye). Iritis, an immune disease of the eye with pain and blurred vision, can occur by itself or as part of other immune diseases. In lupus patients, studies have shown peony and mung-bean extracts can reduce flare ups to 3%. When compared to standard anti-inflammatory medications, such as steroids, in patients with allergic reactions (itchy skin rash from allergies to drugs, exposures, etc.), the remission rate was 48%. But with peony alone, it was 73%.

Recently, we have gained a better understanding as to what happens to the individual cells during inflammation, helping us to understand nutrient remedies. We reviewed the initial sentry cell uptake of the foreign invader, the recruiting of the "T" and "B" cells for disposal, and the inflammatory chemicals causing redness and swelling, which leads us to stage four. Anything adversely affecting our cells here, e.g., free radicals, will force the cell to liberate inside itself NFkB (nuclear factor kappa beta), hooking onto the DNA, so the cell can then respond. Basically, it tells the nucleus of the cell how to react and survive, which is called, "transcriptor."

This then leads us to another concept of chronic inflammation linked to organ dysfunction, and, over time, cancer. At MD Anderson Cancer Hospital in Houston, the Cytokine Laboratory believes 85% of all cancers result from chronic inflammation. So, if you follow this logic, preventing and treating chronic inflammation, more specifically the NFkB, will eliminate 85% of all cancers. This same laboratory recommended curcumin (turmeric), a curry food-extract, a blocker of NFkB, as the answer. Many times, I will use the curcumin in conjunction with resveratrol to enhance the anti NFkB effect and thereby avoid a down-the-road cancer.

How the Mechanisms Work

Oxidation, free radicals, and inflammation mechanisms should not be dismissed lightly. Knowing how they work, when to treat them, and in what context is essential.

The first and most important one is oxidation. I discussed earlier what free radicals (electron deficient) are, and how antioxidants (electron donors) are necessary to neutralize them. These free radicals result from any chemical reaction in the body using oxygen. So, you can imagine the complexity and enormity of this, especially in the lungs where oxygen is being taken in directly. Also, a free radical known as ROS (reactive oxygen species) is particularly bad. We will discuss this later in the book. The converse of this is also true, anything that neutralizes it is a very effective antioxidant.

In summary, by supplying enough antioxidants, the evil empire of oxidation could be preempted. Cell replication and function would then occur normally.

The next important mechanism is anti-inflammatory. Inflammation is a normal body's reaction to many things, from trauma to serious infections. Without it, you could not survive. But when inflammation becomes exaggerated or chronic, it can lead to scarring, organ dysfunction, or abnormal cell reproduction, and then on to cancer. Many examples of chronic inflammation exist as risk factors for the development of cancer, such as esophagitis (esophageal cancer), colitis (colon cancer), cholecystitis (inflammation of gall bladder), and cancer of the gall bladder. These changes are often mediated through chemicals in the body and can be treated, such as NFkB, cytokines, or leukotrienes. Theoretically, by blocking these chemicals, the short- and long-term effects of chronic inflammation can be avoided.

Methylation is something we hear very little of unless we are attending a biochemistry class, but that is changing because of its ability to prevent cancer. We first became aware of its relevancy in giving pregnant women folate and vitamin B supplements to prevent congenital and spinal cord defects.

NO (nitric oxide) is a gas found in blood vessels, but more specifically the endothelial lining cells. (Note: This is different from the gas you get at the dentist's office.) The inner lining of blood vessels releases this gas, causing blood-vessel dilation and increasing blood flow, a very good thing. Nutritional therapies can improve this and may dramatically affect blood flow.

The word hormone is perhaps the most misused word. More money is made illegitimately from hormones than any other nutritional supplement, so knowing how they work is fundamental. Nutritional supplements, like certain drugs, not only will replace them but block, deplete, or enhance them depending on what you want to do. This is a great example of bioengineering and is directly linked to optimal health.

Enzymes in our bodies are responsible for many good things, including digestion, energy creation, and detoxification, among others. Their cousin, coenzymes, are also involved with many of the same reactions. They only help or move reactions along, but are not part of the reaction itself. Basically, they stand by and help, as it were, but are very useful. Don't be fooled with slick marketing techniques, using the moniker "enzymes" to sell something. It does not necessarily mean it is good for you.

Immune function is becoming increasingly important, not only with nutritional therapy but also within medicine itself. In fact, it has become the number one emphasis in preventing and treating cancer. Increasing or decreasing immune function can be manipulated depending on what we want to achieve, since either state can cause negative consequences.

Genetics is truly the field of the future. With bioengineering, you are looking at treating congenital diseases, and changing the course of many other chronic ones, such as diabetes and heart disease. Once the genetic defect is found, the gene can be enhanced for the good ones, or decreased for the bad. For example, if you have the genes for heart disease from your parents, which we can measure, you will need to be very aggressive in getting rid of any risk factors (changing diet, not smoking, exercise). Nutritional therapies will not change the genetics, but you need only change their affects.

Another aspect is cell division. They go through phases from normal cell division to slightly abnormal cell division to cancer cell division. Cells normally die once they reach the end of their life spans, keeping their actual numbers in the normal range. If cells live shorter or longer than normal, disease states occur, such as cancer and leukemia. These all can be manipulated with the use of drugs, nutritional therapies, or both.

Bacteria cover our entire bodies and populate our gastrointestinal tracts. For the most part, we live as good neighbors with them; some even protect us from the bad bacteria. This whole scenario of flora, a concept we will address later when we discuss prebiotics and probiotics, mandates the balance of the good ones over the bad ones. You will never be bacteria-free, and this is a good thing.

The last mechanism involves the concept of receptors. For certain chemicals in our bodies to work, e.g., hormones, they must be taken up by a receptor, like a baseball in a mitt. Once captured, their affect is then mediated. Unless the ball is in the mitt, no response will occur, even if blood levels are normal. This, too, can be influenced by nutrients.

Knowing When and How to Use Nutritional Therapies

Nutritional therapies' usage is unique in one way, but standard in another. The standard usage is to prescribe them when indicated. For example, when a patient has hypertension, a specific medication to lower it is prescribed. Another usage would have to do with patients with no demonstrable medical problem, e.g., hypertension, but nutrients are used to maintain one's health. I call this 'general medical care.' As a corollary, creating an 'antioxidant bank account,' or buildup of antioxidants, will also prevent any process or disease affecting you without your awareness. You could say it's a voluntary preventative against death.

Supplements should be used on a curve. Meaning, if the illness is mild, then it is treated with smaller amounts of supplements (you don't want to shoot a mouse with an elephant gun). But, if severe, more may be necessary. They can also be used in tandem with standard medical care, not as a replacement. It really is the same as prescribing medications in smaller doses, and only a few medications with benign diseases, but using higher doses and many drugs with severe diseases. This book lists useful nutrients and explains their use and how they work.

We all must enter the world of nutrients without being misled by claims of efficiency or costs. There are two dimensions or portals. Let me walk you through them.

The first portal opens to with John Q. Citizen, who has no existing medical problems (prevent medicine). How can he stay healthy and at the same time prolong his life? I've already reviewed the physiology, but we need to put it together in a pragmatic way. John first must realize nutrients are not magic bullets, but rather add-ons to a good diet, exercise, and a lack of bad habits. Without this tandem, the nutrients will only be of marginal value. But add nutrients to this equation, and they can be a powerful tool, doing exactly what they are intended to do.

We are talking here about the general medical care category often mentioned in the context of some nutrients. Having said so, John Q needs to ask, "What nutrients are necessary to maintain my metabolic engines and keep them running?" With John Q, who is passing through the first portal as an unencumbered, uncomplicated, well patient, I first look at his family history as a starting point in evaluating what he needs as far as nutrition, nutrients, and supplements. Factoring in family history, plus what we know about antioxidants, the most common causes of death, and John Q's life style, I can then decide what his options are. If heart disease or cancers are important risk factors, then he should take nutrients to prevent the problem. If John Q smokes or drinks alcohol, I would factor in lung, heart, and liver disease to the equation of what nutrients are needed to prevent them.

The second portal reveals John Q has a recognized medical problem that needs to be addressed (event medicine), whereas the nutrients are then tailored specifically to the problems, along with the medications he is taking. (At the end of this book, you will find a glossary of diseases with recommended nutrients in all their glory; a ready reference for you.) In this case, I would start with the disease and then move forward in conjunction with John's doctor's approval. If his doctor is unaware of the implications, I would then recommend he find someone who knows and is willing to aggressively tackle his case.

Warning: Be wary of advice offered by vitamin and nutrition stores selling nutrients and supplements. Their interest in selling may preempt their interest in your wellbeing. Recall the aforementioned University of Alabama study illustrating their inconsistent recommendations?

The key here is to tailor the nutrients to the disease, and if you follow the guidelines in this book, you will benefit with little risk. Dosing, since it is unregulated, will depend on the brand label, medical advice, or both. The better brands are more expensive but standardized. It's best to research and analyze what you're getting, then make an informed decision.

Frequently Asked Questions:

1. Do all nutrients work? Some but not all nutrients can be used safely alone, along with standard

medical therapy. The information presented in the book, compiled over many years of study and from the experience being gleaned from their use on my patients, is exactly what I teach to my pharmacy students. Don't believe for a minute that all nutrients are good.

2. What about claims? Since nutrients are not controlled by the FDA (U.S. Food and Drug Administration), benefits have not been standardized. Claims can vary from living forever, to growing hair, to curing cancer, even enlarging your penis, so you must be especially vigilant since false claims are rampant. Beware of any claims that seem "too good to be true" and especially unsubstantiated claims made on the Internet or by celebrities. Even today, the TV doctor shows are an extension of this parade of "buy me."

3. What about doses? Determining the proper dose can be a real problem. For example, if you take penicillin, the dose would be standardized to make sure it is therapeutic no matter what brand you choose. This is not true of nutrients, so there are a few simple rules. Listen to your physician's advice, buy a good brand, and follow the directions. A good example of what not to do is buying DHEA (dehydroepiandrosterone) from a grocery or wholesale store. What you are buying is a cheap yam extract and only converts to DHEA in rats. If you are a rat, then it might work, but it doesn't in humans. And, the dose may be affected by what you eat or drink, even milk or grapefruit juice. The responsibility of knowing the interactions and contraindications rests with your physician. There are some exceptions, like with lycopene, where the dose is

15 mg/day, or vitamin C where the recommended dose for women is 2000 mg/, and for men 3000 mg/day. You will also find misconceptions concerning certain nutrients and the drug Coumadin (a blood thinner), where the bleeding concern still exists. You will hear of bleeding problems with EPA (omega-3 oils) or vitamin E; *not* true. I repeat again this crucial advice: consult your physician.

4. What's the difference between herbs and enzymes? The course I teach in the pharmacy school is called "Herbal Medicine," a blatant misnomer. It really should be called "Nutritional Therapies" since it encompasses not only herbs but vitamins, minerals, enzymes, and other chemical substances with nutrient value.

Herbal remedies come from herbs used mostly for cooking. You will see herbs like rosemary and oregano used in conjunction with other nutrient remedies since their actions tend to be small, whereas vitamins, enzymes, and coenzymes are very distinct and powerful chemicals. Trace elements are mostly found in multi-vitamin preparations, except for selenium and chromium, which can have profound influences with cancer and diabetes mellitus respectively. For the most part, selenium and chromium are used individually.

5. How do we use them? It depends on the indications and the portal you are in. Ayurvedic ones (from India) like curcumin (turmeric) may be obtained by consuming a diet rich in curry. I outline how best to use and consume green tea because it is easier to understand the complexities of dietary consumption versus supplements (equivalent doses, etc.). Tinctures, teas, powders, and others are again discussed

with each nutrient since they are all different. For example, vitamin E is better in a cold-pressed powder, but that's not how we take it here in the U.S. Convenience has a price!

6. What about organic? In some cases, "natural" may cost you more and have little advantage. Then again, many people choose to buy organic because they want to avoid pesticide- and hormone-laden, foods. I explain marketing schemes under the umbrella of natural, organic, and free range under its relevant nutrient. Another technique companies use is to rebrand something to make it more appetizing. For example: Chilean sea bass is really the Patagonia tooth fish; it's not from Chile or even a bass! Which one would you prefer?

7. How important is synthetic and soluble? Important aspects of each nutrient are discussed, whether they are natural, synthetic, digestible, polar or nonpolar, fat or water soluble. Multi-vitamins are given a separate category since they may represent an actual hazard for the consumer and are a major marketing rip-off as well. You will be very surprised about the information I provide here. Solubility, very important, is discussed with each nutrient, such as water or fat soluble, stanols and sterols, and how to purchase. Synthetic versus non-synthetic can be extremely important, as with vitamin E, and will be explained in detail.

8. What about misinformation? Most misinformation is purposeful; someone is trying to sell you something. It may sound good, but has no medical benefit and is a waste of your hard-earned money. Southeast Asia has provided us with many clues about nutrients since people

from that region tend to live longer than Westerners. Cancer risks there, especially of the breast, prostate, and uterus, are much lower, along with a dramatic decrease in heart disease. Because our cultures are diverse, drinking five to twenty cups of green tea every day will not work in the United States, but taking green-tea supplements is feasible. The ultimate success will depend on you taking them in adequate amounts. Herbal teas are all caffeine free, an added advantage.

9. What about kidney or liver disease? The excretion (elimination from the body) of nutritional supplements needs to be considered, but to a lesser extent than regular drugs. Adjusting the dose up or down depends on the recommendation of your physician, who can measure levels in your blood. The dosing would, therefore, depend on how bad the liver or kidneys are.

10. What is a good price and where should I buy them? The cheapest are generally the worst, and I strongly recommend you *not* buy them. Go to a reliable nutritional store, or your own doctor, who should have a very intimate knowledge of the best nutrients, can cost compare, and then recommend accordingly. I provide nutrients for my patients in my practice and through the Internet based on that premise. Any purchase, regardless, must be researched for quality along with competitive pricing. The shelf life, like any other food, medicine, or nutrient, needs to be verified, too. Once expired, it can lose its potency and become ineffective. Lastly, make sure you store all medications and nutrients in a cool, dark room — *not* the bathroom; in a warm,

moist environment they degrade quicker. Some keep theirs in the refrigerator.

Our website can provide you with additional important information: www.YourGoodHealthFL.com.

Part of understanding nutrients is following recommended general guidelines. Let me give you an example, a true story of what not to do. A new patient who was feeling well wanted a complete history and physical exam. In the history, I learned she was taking nutrients, and she brought them in for me to review. She promptly gave me four plastic boxes containing *seventy* different bottles. I went through *all* of them. Forty-five minutes later, I had only found seven with any value. She was needlessly spending $450 per month. Why?

Her story is not unusual, though maybe not to this degree. The underlying theme here is she was profoundly interested in nutrient therapy and had been duped by advertising and misinformation. As ridiculous as it seems, this scenario occurs every day. That's why what I am presenting here is vital. Tailor your nutrients like you tailor drugs. You don't take digitalis unless you have heart disease, so why would everyone be on the same nutrients?

Misconceptions

One of the biggest misconceptions has to do with age. When the Lord was creating man, he decided to use age as a biological parameter for our needs, whether nutritional, sexual, or what have you. Then people began to think 'more is better.' Well, neither the human body nor our lives are that simple, so we need to dismiss using more with age for nutritional therapy. True, with gender and age there are some important considerations.

Pre-menopausal women (before menopause) need 1200 mg of calcium daily; post-postmenopausal (after menopause) 1500 mg/day. In addition, they will need vitamin D3 (5000 i.u./day), boron, and strontium to ward off osteoporosis. Also, once women go through menopause, their incidence of heart disease, the number one-killer of women in the USA, is the same as men, making it an important consideration in women's overall care. Beyond this, regarding age, there are no miracle "dial-ups." Forget about marketing techniques using age to lure you in.

One caveat to this aging criterion does pertain to growing older per se. You don't want to get old before your time. People over age fifty may embrace the aging process in general and want guidance. Here, of course, risk factors need to be sorted out and dealt with by your doctor, but DNA considerations — biogenics and hormone levels — need to be looked at. Under general medical care, there are suggestions having to do with acetyl-L-carnitine and lipoic acid for biogenics (to be discussed later). Also, blood levels of DHEA, growth hormone, and testosterone levels need be done; to be replaced if low.

How Do You Know if Something More is Needed?

Why do people go to a particular physician? You need to ask yourself that question; your life may depend on it. A well-trained doctor with years of clinical experience and good people skills is what I prefer. Once you have a trustworthy physician, you need to realize, and your doctor, too, that he or she is in the advice business.

When they prescribe medication, order a test, or refers you to other doctors, they have weighed all the benefits and risks for you and then considers this to be the best course of action. *Not* doing what they have suggested is riskier, in his opinion, than following orders.

Many times, it is a matter of degree. This is where training and experience come in handy. For example, a patient comes in with a blood pressure of 180/120. There is no way nutritional therapy would be sufficient. You can't shoot an elephant with a B-B gun! It is exactly the same for a cholesterol of 300. A nutritional remedy will not be sufficient alone, so medication along with nutrients may be the answer.

Don't entrench yourself with nutrient therapy only; it may put you at risk. Let the doctor you have picked help as he sees fit.

Exercise

Most medical experts agree exercise can be a powerful tool for a longer more vibrant and fulfilling life. What are some effective ways of exercising? Let me start by saying jogging is out and should not be done. Here's a question for you: Who benefits more, someone who jogs one mile or someone who walks a quick-paced one mile? The answer is the same, they both have equal benefit, but jogging, over time, wears out your knees and hips and causes high levels of free-radical damage to the lungs related to lung fibrosis. The only benefit to jogging is it gets you there quicker.

Another key is to mix weight training with isometrics (to elevate your heart rate). You can do both with power walking — walking at a pace brisk enough to get your heart rate up along with light weights (one-to-five pounds), hand held, not ankle weights that can put too much torque on your ankles, knees, and hips, and doing arm movements (nothing jerky; purposeful controlled up-down, back and forth, overhead, and pressed back) while walking.

I play tennis and walk as much as I can and lift weights twice a week. Three times weekly is plenty. Remember, if lifting weights, you need to do three sets of twelve-to-fifteen repetitions with each exercise to achieve maximum benefit, and don't forget to exercise both upper and lower body muscles.

By living by the "holy trinity of medicine" — exercising moderately, eating properly, and getting good medical care with nutrient supplication — you will have a winning combination for a long, healthy life. You need to do all three to be blessed with good health; eliminating any one of them will undermine your success.

Vegans/Vegetarians

In my experience, a very common misconception is that vegetarians are significantly healthier than non-vegetarians. Granted, you are not eating saturated fat and your weight is probably down, but you may not be receiving enough omega-3 and -7 oils, carnitine, CLA (conjugated linoleic acid), calcium, vitamin D3 and B12, which puts you at risk for the very things you are trying to avoid. If you are a vegetarian, you need to replace these nutrients in adequate amounts.

A recent study of normal-weight vegetarians demonstrated they were at three times the risk of heart disease due to these deficiencies. Alert your physician of your vegetarian lifestyle. He can then measure your blood levels and replace what's needed in appropriate amounts. Just because you look like a stick does not make you healthier.

Diabetic Health-conscious Individuals

If you are a diabetic and/or health conscious, two things need to be addressed: fruit and high fructose corn syrup. Fruit, a mainstay in the Mediterranean diet, has, for sure, a nutritional value, especially with the fiber, polyphenols, vitamins, and minerals. But the dark side of fruit is it contains fructose. A fructose molecule in the body is broken down to sugar (glucose), an absolute no-no when it comes to diabetes. You would be surprised how many diabetics eat fruit to an extreme, thinking it is healthy. My rule with diabetics and obesity is one fruit a day *only*. High fructose corn syrup needs to be sought out on *all* labels and the products never bought or, if in your cupboard or refrigerator, thrown away — diet drinks, ketchup, BBQ sauce, and other condiments, baked beans, flavored waters, etc. It is especially highly processed products from corn that have been linked to diabetes, heart disease, and cancer. If you are a diabetic or obese, check all labels and avoid it at all costs.

Also, avoid MSG and partially hydrogenated vegetable oils found in most pre-cooked and packaged foods.

One last thing, we now know fats are not the bad guys in causing heart disease, diabetes, and cancer but rather carbohydrates are the "evil empire." I will discuss this in more detail later, and how the insulin surges brought on by carbs is the common denominator.

Fatigue

Taking something for granted can be a major mistake in both medicine and in life in general. For example, chronic fatigue syndrome is very common, distressing, and many times overlooked or dismissed by the medical community at large. Now thought to be due to the Epstein-Barr and/or the Cytomegalic virus (both herpes viruses), there are other valid reasons to be concerned. Currently, there is data to suggest the EB virus is also linked to lupus and a blood cancer called lymphoma. The Cytomegalic virus has also been linked to pancreatitis and immune deficiencies that can lead to certain other blood cancers. If you have chronic fatigue, have your doctor get blood levels for these viruses and treat them. My choice? Fucoidans, branched chain amino acids, lipoic acid, reishi, cistanche, and ginseng, which will increase immunity against the viruses and increase energy. Don't let your doctor dismiss this disease as it is a recognized entity with long-term consequences, such as cancer.

A Note on Inflammation

In medicine, things change on almost a daily basis. We're now talking about quantum inflammation, the key to just about every major disease. TNF (Tumor Necrosis Factor) is related to diseases like RA (rheumatoid arthritis), IBS (inflammatory bowel syndrome), and psoriasis. DMARDS (disease modifying anti-rheumatic drugs) are methotrexate, cyclosporine, and cytoxan to treat them. These acronyms demonstrate chronic inflammatory diseases with new single target drugs. TNF, along with the interleukins, are the most commonly mentioned inflammatory chemicals.

Mitochondria

One of the most exciting new concepts is mitochondria. As the energy producing (gas tank) organelle in every cell of our body (2-2000 per/cell), it's the reason why the cell can function normally and reproduce itself; a direct link to aging. As we get older, they decrease in number, making their maintenance and growth a paramount importance. Acetyl-L-carnitine, branched amino acids, lipoic acid, and CoQ10 are great ways to revitalize them; labeling them necessary for anti-aging purposes, too.

The New Understanding

It would be wise to look to the future. In 1994, Laurie Garrett's book, *The Coming Plague,* outlined in specific detail how resistant bacteria would gradually take over and kill all of us. Scary! But another plague is already here: electronics.

In the early 1990s, La Quinta high school in California opened a new state-of-the-art facility (wireless). Within a very short period of time, both teachers and students became sick with vague medical problems, and eventually, over years, equated to a cancer risk of about 60%. It was eventually linked to EMFs, a form of radiation created by the state-of-the-art electronics. Since then, we have added routers, wi-fi, compact florescent bulbs, cell phones, laptop computers, etc. — more EMFs.

The topic of brain tumors related to cell phones keeps raising its head and has been established by several European studies, and yet we cannot see the plague. Why did Steve Jobs, the father of laptops, die of an unusual pancreatic tumor? Is it a coincidence, just bad luck, or a manifestation of the coming plague?

We have surrounded ourselves with electronics leaking radiation in the form of electromagnetic fields. These fields, like gamma radiation, destroy DNA, pre-empting the normal cell division in our bodies, leading to aging and cancer mutations. Speculation exists of three scenarios where electromagnetic fields cause human disease. One is the summation of all of them — computers, flat-screens, cell phones, tablets, i-Pods, and all other electrical devices — made even worse if you live in a tight sub-division and/or near power lines, or spend the majority of your time in a particular area/room of your home on or near those devices (office, entertainment/recreation room), making it dirty, or full of electrical fog. The second results from our power companies supplying our electricity. AC (alternating current) does not allow the magnet fields to clear to an endpoint. It goes back and forth instead of clearing and accumulates. The last is an allergy some people have to the fields.

In my medical practice, I have been seeing many young men with low "T" syndrome (low testosterone). I attribute this to the plague of electrical energy. My advice is to avoid electrical fields as much as you can, such as cell phones, especially in pants pockets or close to the body, and make sure the battery is facing out. Don't put your laptop on your lap, get that router out from under your desk, and turn off the wi-fi when not using it.

Diet

The last cog in the wheel of good health is diet. Depending on your medical problems, perhaps diabetes or heart failure, special diets are required; the garden-variety diet (pardon the pun) is debatable. Head-to-head studies have been done over a long period of time and the winner is the Adkins's diet. It not only takes off the most weight, but keeps it off the best and improves blood tests (cholesterol). The reason is the cutting of the carbs, not the fats, which results in better outcomes.

For almost fifty years, we have been told fats are the bad guys. This is far from the truth. Numerous recent studies have shown that increased carbs have been linked to an increase in cancer, presumably because of the insulin surges they produce. Insulin, a growth factor, is believed to be the reason. The South Beach diet and the Glycemic Indexes are off-shoots of the same principle, limiting the amount of insulin being produced. My choice would be the Adkin's diet for people who are overweight, followed by the Mediterranean diet, which is ideal once your BMI (body mass index) is lower than twenty-five. The Mediterranean diet combines fruits, vegetables, and meats along with red wine and olive oil making it a close second to the Adkins's diet but much more palatable over a long period of time.

Nutritional therapies need to be followed in the context of our cultural differences, diet, exercise, and proper medical care. In my opinion, patients are best served by doctors who focus on preventative care, are nutritionally oriented, and who don't immediately reach for their prescription pads.

Glycemic Index

The Glycemic Index is a concept involving carbohydrates wherein all carbs are not considered bad. Carbs are graded by absorption rates, with the worst or the fastest being sugar with an index score of 100. Sugar is bad due to its quick absorption, causing an insulin surge. Any carb above fifty-five is not good for you for this reason. But the lower ones, those absorbed much slower, are not only *not* bad for you but *good* for other reasons. Just as an aside, marinating food with vinegar prior to cooking, and/or adding beans to the meal will also decrease absorption time, thereby decreasing the insulin surge associated with it. Consuming beans with every meal, if possible, is a great idea if you do not have issues with gas and bloating. Incidentally, Beano does help relieve this gas problem. Beans' slow absorption and decreased insulin levels will help you manage and/or prevent diabetes, heart disease, and cancer.

Chapter Two

Muscle, Brain, and Blood Vessels

Our blood vessels are the main highways carrying oxygen and nutrients to our cells so they can function normally. The venous system then returns the blood to be re-oxygenated and removes waste products from the cells. Muscles are the mechanics of movement, but smooth muscles also help us digest our food, and the brain is the computer system keeping everything coordinated, using a wiring mechanism much like in our homes.

Carnitine

Principally found in our body's muscle tissue (striated and cardiac), carnitine's main function is to build and repair it. How does it do this?

1. Helps transport ATP (adenosine triphosphate) from the mitochondria of our cells that make energy, so the cell may perform optimally and reproduce.

2. Also helps maintain cardiac enzymes, enabling the heart to recover from exercise or exertion, and supports left ventricular function, increasing our strength. The left ventricle is responsible for the amount of blood leaving the heart, E.F, (ejection fraction) and supplying the rest of the body. This measurement, determined by a heart

echo exam, needs to be over 50%; less would indicate a serious underlying heart problem.

3. Has been shown to decrease the aging in rats by 34% by blocking oxidation and decreasing body fat.
4. Increases bone density (preventing osteoporosis) and decreases age-related muscle weakness.

The indications for carnitine's usage include: muscle disorders from heart to skeletal — fibromyalgia, polymyositis, congestive heart failure, post heart attacks, osteoporosis, and cardiomyopathy — to general medical care. It will also enhance exercise potential. The dosage has not really been established, so buy a good brand and follow the recommended dose. Note: more is not always better and could be harmful or even fatal.

Acetyl-L-Carnitine

Found in the brain and muscle, with the former being the most important. Acetyl-L-Carnitine does three important things when it comes to the brain:

1. Stimulates brain cells to grow (brain plasticity).
2. Releases and synthesizes a chemical that helps make the brain work better.
3. Releases dopamine and binds the dopamine receptors integral to nerve transmission. Helps the brain function normally and repair itself. Lastly, it may also help the brain be less susceptible to injury.
4. Prevents mitochondrial damage and helps regenerate new mitochondria in the brain, an important new concept in avoiding the aging process.

5. The dose will again depend on the quality of the brand you buy with indications including TIA (transient ischemia attacks), brain dysfunctions of less than twenty-four hours seen in recovering stroke patients, and in early dementias, such as Alzheimer's disease. It is also for heart disease prevention and general medical care as it pertains to aging. When I use acetyl-L-carnitine for specific brain problems, I almost always use it in combinations with gingko, lipoic acid, PS (phosphatidylserine), gastrodin, magnesium threonate, taurine, and vinpocetine.

Carnosine

An amino acid, carnosine is found in nerves, muscles, and eye tissue. It diminishes in time, with aging, to 63% of normal. It is found in red meat with an average of 250 mg in a meal, but the enzyme carnosinase in our bodies rapidly degrades it, so we do not benefit much from a standard meal. However, by oversupplying it in the form of supplements, therapeutic levels can be achieved. It works by suppression of oxidation and glycation (we will discuss this shortly).

1. Neutralizes the ROS molecules, the real super-duper bad guys.
2. Prevents AGE (advanced glycation end) products, sugar molecules, from hooking onto proteins, like our DNA, and deactivating them. With dysfunctional proteins in your DNA, you become very susceptible to other diseases and age rapidly. You see them a lot in diabetics; the wrinkles like the vertical ones around the mouth (smokers are particularly prone to them) are a result of AGE products.

3. Increases the effectiveness of the cardiac muscle by increasing calcium usage in the heart, as does digitalis. For patients with congestive heart failure, it can be very effective.
4. Helps maintain DNA with its superoxide dismutase activity (SOD). Carnosine and catalase are the two strongest antioxidants in the body.
5. Increases the life span of flies by 20-36%. There may be a fair comparison to humans.
6. Decreases arterial plaque and avoids the "double hit" phenomenon of a stroke. Simply put, a double hit means, in the incidence of a stroke, initially, there is not enough blood circulating to the brain. This causes cell death, and when the blood returns, more damage to the brain cells occurs.
7. Decreases oxidative damage from the sun on the cornea, lens, and retina.
8. Indications for usage include: wrinkles, diabetes mellitus, eye problems (cataracts), heart or muscular disorders, and general medical care, with the dose being 1000 mg/day.

Since carnosine is vital to the eyes, a word about macular degeneration is helpful here.

Despite the lack of interest and not caring for nutrient therapies, the standard practice of medicine is now being forced to take notice. Just recently a Medicare publication listed the highest paid doctors with eye-opening results. The highest paid physicians were mostly ophthalmologists. Why would eye doctors be the highest paid? The answer could be they choose to treat macular degeneration with an eye injection (Lucentis) that is required every month and costs $4000 per injection. There is a cheaper one called Avastin at only fifty dollars, but they choose the former. Why? As you will see in chapter nine, other natural alternatives help prevent and treat the same problem, but they all are nutrients.

The macula is responsible for central vision, which, over time, starts to degenerate for various reasons; one being ultraviolet light from the sun. Patients complain about a gradual loss of central vision that sometimes goes unnoticed because it occurs over several years. For example, you can't see someone's face but you can see all the surroundings.

There are two types: a "dry," 90% of the cases, and a "wet," 10%. The latter is by far the most dangerous and about two-thirds of all the severe cases. Oxidation from the sun's radiation causes degeneration in the form of drusen deposits along the choroidal layer of the retina. New blood vessels in this layer leak and replace light-sensitive cells and the retinal pigment lining cells. This also occurs in diabetic retinopathy, along with the leakage, but here the leakage causes a separation of the retinal layers, leading to diabetic blindness. Diabetics need a retinal exam every year by an ophthalmologist to check for this problem, which can be treated with laser therapy before the hemorrhage even occurs. The only way to diagnose is to use an intravenous injection and then observe the retina.

The aging of the retina, due to oxidation and living longer, can only be limited to a certain extent. So, what can we do? Simple things, like wearing a hat with a large brim minimizes light exposure to the eye by 60%, and large sunglasses with wrap-around side protection will also help considerably. Think of the same protection for your children, even the ones in their buggies. And, supplement with carnosine, which also helps prevent cataracts. Lastly, lutein, bilberry, beta carotene and zeaxanthine will help prevent and treat   macular degeneration.

Branched Chain Amino Acids

Branched chain amino acids include: leucine, isoleucine, and valine; all responsible for making new mitochondria, muscle energy, and repair. When absorbed from the gastrointestinal tract, these go directly to muscle tissue for absorption and aren't broken down directly like other food substrates. Once in the cell, they are used for protein production and energy. The more branched chains are studied, the more we learn, and the list of benefits gets longer.

1. Regulates the live-longer gene that resveratrol targets.
2. Increases NOS (nitric oxide synthase that makes nitric oxide), which enlarges the diameter of blood vessels and thus increases blood flow.
3. Compliments pyrrolequinoline (PQQ), quinone, and CoQ10, increase life span in a similar manner as resveratrol and sirtuins through the support of our DNA.
4. Helps form glutamate and a neurotransmitter, gamma butyric acid, expediting brain function and improving thought processes by slowing down the brain.
5. Stimulates mTor, a regulatory signaling protein that helps with protein synthesis and calorie consumption through leptin, the anorectic hormone. More importantly, mTor is a signaling protein for cancer formation in about 80% of

tumors, so this effect may have tremendous benefits in prevention.

Knowing all these actions makes branched chain amino acids' indications self-evident, i.e., general medical care and aging, obesity, metabolic syndrome, and diabetes mellitus, liver, muscle, and heart disease, chronic fatigue, mitochondrial support, cancer prevention, and weight loss. This along with lipoic acid, acetyl-L-carnitine, fucoidans, reishi, cistanche, and ginseng are very effective in treating chronic fatigue syndrome/ fibromyalgia, a common ailment in all age groups. The dosage again depends on the brand.

Pomegranate

Pomegranate was used by the Roman armies for centuries. The active ingredient is polyphenols. The research involved has become immense and impressive.

1. Stimulates the PONS (peroxygenase) receptor located on the high-density lipoprotein, the good cholesterol, molecule. Inhibits LDL (the bad cholesterol) by decreasing the lipid peroxidase. It will actually remove existing plaque from arterial walls (makes you younger).
2. Breaks apart an amino acid that causes heart disease. It turns out the resveratrol in red wine has the same benefit.
3. Prevents advanced glycation products (AGE), and regulates the gene to decrease cholesterol and LDL. Clinical studies have shown pomegranate *decreases* carotid artery thickening by 35% in one year, as compared to a statin medication (like Lipitor) for cholesterol that resulted in a 9% *increase* of carotid thickening.

4. Decreases blood pressure through its blockage of an enzyme that can lead to hypertension, which standard medications do (ACE inhibitors).
5. Ellagic acid (a natural phenol antioxidant found in numerous fruits and vegetables) in it decreases inflammation through its blockage of NFkB.
6. Increases prostacyclin, preventing platelet clumping and possibly heart attacks.
7. Combats weight gain, diabetes, and systemic inflammation. The flower extract enhances gene expression of a fat tissue gene linked to diabetes and heart disease, which regulates cellular response to energy and helps normalize blood sugar levels. The result, it decreases cardiac fibrosis associated with diabetes that causes congestive heart failure.
8. Pomegranate seed oil decreases endothclin-1 and NFkB involved with inflammation.
9. Inhibits an enzyme that converts testosterone to estrogen (and leads to low testosterone syndrome) and blocks 17-beta hydroxysteroid dehydrogenase, which converts a weak estrogen to estradiol, a stronger one that can lead to breast cancer, heart, disease, and diabetes. In men, you can easily see it with their large breasts and small testicles. Problems with a low libido and/or erectile dysfunction could improve greatly.
10. May help prevent cancer by inhibiting VEGF, which provides blood vessels for tumor growth. In addition, both the flower extracts and seed oil have punicic acid, an inhibitor of both estrogen-dependent and independent breast cancer cells. The punicic acid also kills cancer cells by 91% for both breast and prostate cancers.

Not only is the pomegranate fruit itself important for medicinal purposes, but the flower extract and the seed oil have benefits, too, with their own separate chemicals not found in the other areas. Therefore, if you only eat the fruit you will lose the benefits from the other areas.

The dose is again brand related with indications including: heart disease, cancer (breast and prostate), and risk factors for heart disease like coronary artery disease, hyperlipidemia, congestive heart failure, diabetes mellitus, hypertension, low-T syndrome, arthritis, and general medical care.

Everyone should be on it and make sure the supplement has all three: fruit, flower, and seed extract. Of course, don't forget, eat the fruit, too.

Arginine

Arginine is a non-essential amino acid your body can manufacture and is not dietary required.

1. Increases blood flow by releasing nitric oxide from the inner lining of blood vessels.
2. Helps support thinking.
3. May help diabetics by increasing insulin and growth hormones, thereby improving glucose tolerance.
4. Increases exercise tolerance and helps with bladder dysfunction (bladder spasms — going to urinate every thirty minutes).
5. Vasodilates arteries in the penis; can be used like Cialis and Viagra for erectile problems.
6. Because of its dramatic effects, use Arginine with caution for: migraine, depression, and psychosis, autoimmune disease, liver and kidney

disease, and herpes infections susceptible to activation.

The dose is brand determined every twelve hours. Indications include: peripheral vascular disease (decreased blood flow into the legs), sexual dysfunction, diabetes, or any condition requiring vasodilatation (dilation of blood vessels), such as Raynaud's disease. Lastly, research shows bladder dysfunction and brain disease (TIA) may also benefit. It also helps with sensitive teeth where the dentine is too thin.

Passion Flower

When visiting the Grand Canyon, I noticed this pretty little plant, so named because the flower looks like the Passion of Christ with the crown of thorns. The guide told us the plant had been used by the Indians for medicinal purposes for centuries.
1. Affects the central nervous system with a flavonoid active ingredient.
2. Has sedative effects, and many times is used with lavender, valerian, or lemon balm for sleep.
3. Has mild cardiac actions so it may be used with CoQ10 and hawthorn for hypertension.

The dose is brand-directed and its main indication is anxiety.

Mung Bean Extract

The use of mung beans goes back 1500 years in India. As you will see, it does many good things, but our primary emphasis will be on inflammation.

The Chinese have labeled mung bean extract as a "cooling agent" for centuries, and how right they were. When a cell is injured, a biochemical switch releases a store of approximately 150 chemicals that cause inflammation. These can be danger signals to the various organs involved and must be turned off.

1. Mung bean extract along with a green tea polyphenol in concert with their "cooling effect," decreases HMG both in and outside the cells, thus preempting the whole process at the cellular-cytokine level. You can see how in understanding its physiology it can be used with asthma, heart disease, arthritis, cancer prevention, diabetes, and infectious diseases.
2. Very useful in arthritis, bursitis, and tendon problems resistant to standard medications.
3. The active ingredients we find in other things, like passion flower, is used for mild anxiety, and has a cooling effect, too.
4. Lowers blood pressure, and LDL levels (the bad cholesterol) via ACE-inhibiting activity. ACE drugs, incidentally, are very popular HBP (high blood pressure) medications, so it has the same type of activity.
5. Decreases AGE products — sugar molecules that attach to proteins — deactivating them, and preventing the cell from reproducing itself when it becomes aged. That's why diabetics age quickly; the disease affects their blood vessels. Again, you can see these advanced glycation end products by looking in the mirror. If you have vertical wrinkles or lines running up and down from your lip area, then you have increased levels that can be treated with mung bean and carnosine.

6. A Harvard study reported eating mung beans twice weekly decreases breast cancer by 24%. Another study showed consuming mung beans decreased colon cancer rates by 42%. The soluble fiber in them ferments to short chain fatty acids (butyrates), a protector of the DNA in the colon cells and cuts the blood supply to the tumors, hindering grow.
7. Increases amounts of folate, potassium, fiber, and magnesium in it, which may be beneficial for migraines, heart disease, and general cellular metabolism.

You can buy the beans and cook them for all these reasons or take mung bean extract. My patients with inflammatory problems are all on it, along with people at risk for heart disease, diabetes, and cancer (especially colon cancer). The ability of mung beans to help bring down insulin surges cannot be stressed enough since it is related to adult diabetes and cancer, with insulin having these growth-factor qualities.

Zyflamend

Zyflamend is a Chinese concoction of nine phytonutrients (from plants) of an herbal nature, containing mostly Cox-2 activity. Cox-2 is an enzyme system that mediates inflammation, principally in joints leading to arthritis. Many drugs are directed at Cox-2 activity, like Celebrex, Voltaren, Naprosyn, and Arthrotec, and do not affect Cox-1 activity as do Motrin, Advil, and Aleve, which have an increased GI track bleeding risk. Zyflamend came to fame thanks to Columbia University, an unlikely source, with its work on preventing prostate cancer, where it found Zyflamend can prevent cancer by 30%. It recommends any patient at risk for cancer of the prostrate (family history or Vietnam agent-orange exposure) should be on it. Active ingredients include:

1. Holy Basil, a Cox-2 inhibitor.
2. Turmeric — Cox inhibitor and enhances the polyphenols in green tea.
3. Ginger — Cox inhibitor that can be used alone for the treatment of arthritis.
4. Green tea — Cox inhibitor and polyphenols.
5. Rosemary — Cox inhibitor.
6. Hu hang — Cox activity with high levels of resveratrol.
7. Chinese goldthread and barberry — Cox inhibitors.
8. Oregano — decreases fluid retention, like a diuretic.
9. Scutellaria or Baikal Skullcap — Cox inhibitor.
1. Indications include the prevention and treatment of prostate cancer and arthritis. I find this a very useful adjunct to patients who have arthritis and can't take or don't want the standard arthritis medications with the dose brand-directed.

Gastrodin

When I read the original reports regarding gastrodin, I thought of a movie Sean Connery made a few years ago called *Medicine Man*. He was a physician investigator in the Amazon looking for a cure for cancer in an orchid. The orchid turned out to be an innocent bystander, but was a home for an ant colony that was providing the cancer-curing chemicals. Regardless, an orchid led to the cure, just as God had intended, and without it, the ants were just ants. God tries to point us in the right direction, toward color and odors, but most times we ignore it. An orchid, gastrodia elata, with its brilliant color and smell, provides us with a "brain shield," as the Chinese describe it, and, in fact, will grow the brain. The mechanisms are also interesting and make sense, leading us into other areas of treatment.

Its most important action is to regenerate brain cells through brain cell reorganization and activating genes — brain plasticity.

1. Activates 20% of the genes linking one brain cell to another and protein 1, regenerating new neurons. It basically, through genetics, turns on methods that improve the wiring of the brain, memory, and thinking and make it grow.
2. Improves blood blow to the brain, allowing all these things to happen. In stroke patients, it has been shown to improve blood flow by 96%. Cardiac by-pass patients generally have a 30% memory loss called "pump-head syndrome," which is reduced to 9% when gastrodin is used pre-op.
3. Switches on other genes that decrease the production of amyloid and tau proteins in our brains. Of course, I'm speaking of Alzheimer's disease, making gastrodin an *obvious* use in these patients, especially in their early stages.
4. Decreases excitatory impulses and inflammation of the brain seen in these patients, as well as seizures. It does so by decreasing glutamic acid levels and increasing transmission of gamma butyric acid levels in the brain. It then switches on misfolded protein responses to destroy the normal ones.
5. Improves migraine headaches by decreasing excitatory impulses, especially when magnesium

is added to the therapy. Magnesium seems to enhance gastrodin effects by increasing neurotransmissions rates. Subsequently, a combination of the two is optimal.

2. The indications are clear for any brain dysfunction, especially if dementia is a part of it; acute things, like neurological dysfunction lasting less than twenty-four hours and completed strokes. For chronic problems like Alzheimer's disease, Parkinsonism, and Lewy-Body dementia, it could be equally effective. For seizure patients, it can be a reasonable add-on to the standard seizure treatments in patients who are not responding as well, and those with break-through seizures and, finally, migraines with magnesium.

Magnesium Threonate

For years we have known the importance of magnesium for brain function — migraine headaches, seizures — but to get this heavy ion into the central nervous system (brain) could not be accomplished because too much of an oral dose caused diarrhea. MIT (Massachusetts Institute of Technology) found hooking it onto threonate increased brain levels by 15%, which doesn't sound like much but is astronomical! In therapeutic doses, it increased brain plasticity and improved memory.

1. With calcium, opens ionic channels triggering nerve transmission.
2. Increases NMDN (N methyl D glutamate) receptors for memory by 52%.
3. Triggers "Bouton" (synapse release of ions) for memory.

Clinical studies have shown all kinds of memory improved — short term, long term, spatial, and pattern completion. Rapid improvement was seen in Alzheimer's patients and there may be some benefit for PTSD. The dose is 150 mg, two-three times a day.

Gingko

Gingko Biloba comes from an oriental tree.

Studies have shown:

1. Increases availability of oxygen to brain cells.
2. Decreases free-radical activity in the brain.
3. In stroke patients, decreases brain damage by 60%.
1. Indications include any brain dysfunction, at the recommended dose. One caveat: it must be used early in the problem and is not indicated for moderate to severe problems.

Phosphatidylserine (P.S.)

Derived from soy and found naturally in cell membranes. We find, with aging, as with many important chemicals in our body, the levels go down, and as a result, the brain starts to age.

Actions include:

1. Increases energy in the brain cells, stimulating memory, concentration, word choice, and learning.
2. Maintains brain-cell membrane integrity and plasticity.

3. Increases choline levels in the brain, and, in turn, nerve transmission.

The dose is 100 mg twice daily, and the indications include any brain dysfunction.

Vinpocetine

An extract from the periwinkle plant. Small amounts are absorbed and processed in the liver, but most tissues absorb it directly.

1. In the brain, it allows oxygen distributions into the brain's cells, and to the hemoglobin itself, thereby increasing oxygenation and use of sugar in the brain, causing vasodilatation and improving circulation.
2. Double-blind controlled studies showed increased cognitive function.
3. Improves memory and attention.
4. Seems to benefit tinnitus, or ringing in the ears, a symptom of inner-ear disease, and bladder spasms with frequent urination.
5. This, along with PS and Huperzine, can be used for peripheral neuropathy with burning in the legs.

The dosage is brand-directed with indications including: dementias, TIA, strokes, Alzheimer's, tinnitus (ringing in the ears), peripheral neuropathies, and bladder spasms.

Taurine

The last to the "brain party" is taurine, an amino acid that slows things down by turning down the autonomic nervous system. The autonomic nervous system runs "automatically," — heart, breathing, gastrointestinal tract, bladder, etc. — to stay alive.

1. Activates "sleeping" or "hibernating" brain-stem cells and increases brain cellular activity.
2. Animal studies have shown it increases brain cells in the hippocampus areas, the memory centers.
3. Early clinical studies report Parkinsonism's patients improve 'knowing' Levodopa (Sinemet), a drug used for Parkinsonism, will lower brain taurine levels.
4. Helps lower blood pressure by turning off the sympathetic nervous system.

The dose is brand directed, but it seems every day there are more uses for taurine. Besides brain dysfunction, most heart problems will benefit as well.

Chapter Three

The Oils

Introduction

Your body, as any fine machine, needs to be "oiled up." If you don't, it will eventually rust and stop working. This chapter will help explain how to oil these tiny machines to keep them running for a long time.

EPA Oils

In the 1980s, Dr. Paul Brunwald at Harvard University was the first reputable authority to promulgate the idea of the EPA (omega-3 fish oils) as a remedy for certain disorders. Since then, there have been reams of scientific evidence demonstrating his correctness. But EPA (eicosatetraenoic acid) is only one-half the story, with DHA (docosahexaenoic acid), the other half. These omega-3 oils are found in fish like salmon, sardines, and anchovies from northern waters. The first real evidence of their effectiveness was a medical study done on cultural groups showing Eskimos, despite their high-fat diet, had a low heart attack rate. This paradox was explained by the fish oils (EPA, DHA) protecting them from the fat they ate. Unfortunately, our diet is devoid of the omega-3 oils and loaded with omega-6 oils, like trans-fatty acids, which are bad for us. Omega-3 oils are found everywhere in our bodies, including the brain and all cell membranes, with 100 billion brain neurons having approximately 8% of our total body weight in omega-3 oils.

Recent studies have elucidated just how important the EPA oils are in and by themselves with post heart-attack patients. Absolute blood levels translated to a decreased mortality of 30% if the blood levels were greater than 8%. That means vegetarians and vegans are at greater risk of heart disease since plant sources are low in EPA oils. Even flax seed, walnuts, and canola oil translate to a lower level, and eating farm-raised fish, like tilapia or catfish, fed soy-based grain instead of algae and plankton, have zero EPA oils. That's bad news for people who don't eat meat to prevent heart disease.

EPAs, as mentioned earlier, have a "stop mechanism" dependent on EPA and DHA. So, you should consume both to effectively stop inflammation. And, we now have available a blood tests for the omega-3 oils.

<u>Omega-3</u>

Omega-3 oils:

1. Decreases cholesterol, triglycerides, and LpA particles (lipid particle, also known as "the widow maker," which increases the likelihood of a heart attack by three-to-five times), while increasing the HDL (good cholesterol). If the LpA particle is elevated, the EPA oils with niacin are the only things that will lower it.
2. Increases blood flow and decreases the size of blood-vessel plaque.
3. Decreases the pro-inflammatory chemicals involved with arthritis (decreases inflammation) and with "stop molecules" (i.e. Lipoxins

protections) interrupt on-going inflammation, preventing it from reoccurring.

4. Increases P300 brain waves linked to memory and learning that decrease with age and dementia.

5. Increases immune responses to breast and prostate cancer.

6. Decreases immune response in the GI tract that can be used to treat colitis, such as Crohn's disease and ulcerative colitis.

7. Decreases the risk of age-related macular degeneration.

8. Increases IQ of children, as reported in the *Lancet* journal, by 48%. Stabilizes brain membranes to affect mental problems, such as bipolar, depression, and aggressive behaviors.

9. With its "stop-molecules," it will interrupt any inflammation going on in the body from any source.

10. The dose is between 2-3 g (2,000-3,000 mg) day, taken with food as its fat solubility is absorbed better with transport, just like vitamin D. I advise strongly to get a good brand (you may pay a buck more, but the benefits are greater). Lastly, krill, omega-3 extract, is not as good, unless you are taking the oils for brain function, in which case the krill is better.

The indications for its use follow all this data and includes: general medical care, colitis, arthritis, lipids, coronary artery disease, peripheral artery disease, inflammation, strokes and cerebral insufficiency (TIA), stents post-placement, renal failure, cancer, especially the prevention and treatment of the breast and prostate, PMS and menopause, macular degeneration (prevention and treatment), psoriasis, and mental problems, such as depression, bipolar, and aggressive behavior, even in children.

Krill Oils

Promoted recently, krill oils are found in shrimp-like crustaceans of the Arctic and Antarctic waters. They contain the omega-3 oils, with small amounts of astaxanthin and choline, which do not seem to increase its effectiveness. The ConsumerLab.com gave them a 'thumbs down' due to spoilage and lower amounts of omega-3 oils as advertised in them. Also, there is an environmental concern of depleting krill oil for supplements; it's a marine food essential, sperm whale for example. People with shrimp allergies (iodine) may also react to it. Although recently, there is some evidence with brain considerations — TIA or stroke patients — krill will work better than the standard omega-3 oils.

Flaxseed Oil

The flaxseed itself cannot be digested intact and must be ground up or chewed before consumption. It contains two basic chemicals: 1) plant chemicals — almost identical to human estrogen — to help with breast, prostate, PMS, and menopause, and 2) alpha linoleic acid, of which 20% is converted to an omega-3 oil, its active ingredient.

1. Both will help increase immune-cell function (preventing infections), improve joints (arthritis), and decrease lipids.
2. The Mayo Clinic found, in relation to menopause, four tablespoons per day over six weeks decreased hot flashes by 50%.

Indications include: general health care, cancer prevention, PMS, menopause, and joint pain. Remember, it must be chewed or crushed prior to consumption, and the dose has not been established for certainty. Also, there is some controversy regarding flax seeds and prostate cancer. I would be inclined to not use it if prostate cancer is a concern. Flax seed contains an immense amount of fiber; great for elimination (bowel movements). One tablespoon of flaxseed equals forty cups of broccoli; making it a good remedy for IBS (irritable bowel syndrome) alongside a good probiotic.

Borage Oil

The active ingredient is GLA (gamma linoleic acid), generally used in conjunction with flax oil. It decreases inflammation, mostly in arthritis patients, and the dose is again brand determined. In most cases, I use it with MSM (methysufonylmethane) and glucosamine for the treatment of osteoarthritis. More recently, GLA has been proven to help prevent, and even treat, cancer of the pancreas alongside soy protein, vitamin D, and curcumin.

Dr. Ruth Lupu at the Mayo Clinic has done some amazing work on how GLA can kill cancer cells. If you are at risk with a family history for it, are diabetic, have recurrent pancreatitis, or drink too much alcohol, then I would recommend taking this at the recommended doses per label.

Olive Oil

Primarily considered a nutraceutical (a food with nutrient medical benefit), olive oil has a long history. The ancient Greeks realized its potential and many just drank a glass of olive oil every day. It is an integral part of the Mediterranean diet, making it the best long-term diet to follow.

Olive oil contains two things: 1) Monounsaturated oils- oleic acid, and 2) Polyphenols – typrosol, hydroxy typrosol, and oleuropein.

We know the following about olive oil, but the list gets longer every day:

1. Recent studies show, for diabetes mellitus, olive oil inhibits an enzyme that converts sugar to fat. Oleuropein also prevents the conversion of amylin to TPA (toxic peptide aggregate) that can cause diabetes and cancer of the pancreas.
2. It prevents a normal pancreatic hormone that works with insulin to destroy beta cells, making insulin.
3. Inhibits H. pylori, the bacteria that causes stomach ulcers and gastric cancer.
4. In bone physiology, it decreases calcium loss from bones seen in osteoporosis.
5. In a recent Norwegian study of olive oil with fish oils, it decreased aortic arch plaque (gaining of blood vessels) by 56%. It is believed it does so by decreasing fat build up, increasing good cholesterol, and decreasing triglyceride and bad cholesterol levels.
6. Decreases platelet stickiness, thereby preventing heart attacks, reported *Lancet*, the British Medical Journal.
7. Olive oil can, regarding cancer, interact with signal pathways to prevent cancer and/or its spread, increase cancer cell death, suppress fatty-acid synthase that acts as a cancer suppressor,

and inhibit the invasion by colon and gastric cancer cells.

The dose has not been established, but I recommend using EVOO (Extra Virgin Olive Oil - the darker green the better) as much as possible. Put it on all the food you eat and use it in your cooking. Indications include: the prevention of cancer in general, heart disease and its risk factors, diabetes, general medical care, and osteoporosis. Gastric-ulcer patients should be on a steady diet of it not only to heal an ulcer but also to possibly prevent gastric cancer from H. pylori.

<u>Omega-7</u>

These oils are monounsaturated, compared to the Omega-3 polyunsaturated oils, and have completely different modes of action, even though they sound the same. Omega-7, or palmitoleic acid, signals molecules communicating between fat and muscle tissue; they tell the energy nutrients where to go, making them hormone-like molecules that link distant body tissue to assure maximum energy and storage. Harvard has applied for a patent on it, which tells you how important they are.

1. Perhaps one of the most important benefits of the omega-7 oils is its effectiveness with diabetes. Adult diabetes is on the rise and accounts for many health dollars spent with its many human organ dysfunctions and early death rates. As an internist, I see more diabetics in one day than patients with any other underlying problem. Because diabetics develop heart disease, and all its ramifications, early on, the heart disease gets immediate attention, but the diabetes is the main, underlying problem. The secret here is if you

control the blood sugars, the risks all go away. Simple.

2. Omega-7 oils act much like certain medications: Lipitor (statin) for LDL (bad cholesterol), Lopid for a high triglyceride level or a low HDL level (the good cholesterol), and actos (for diabetes) to lower blood sugar. It has been found to act as three drugs in one.

Here is an itemized list of what they do and you will see overlapping benefits of these three drugs.

Omega-7s:

1. Reduces the bad cholesterol.
2. Increases the good cholesterol.
3. Reduces blood sugar.
4. Reduces insulin resistance.
5. Reduces appetite and, thus, weight.
6. Reduces inflammation.
7. Omega-7s have *no* side effects.

Incidentally, its ability to reduce inflammation is unique here in that it affects the fat tissue directly, the root cause of inflammation. How's that? Fat tissue, specifically large adipocytes, is not just a fat storage area, but is metabolically active, secreting hormones (estrogen), adiponectin, leptin, and TNF, all of which have negative effects. That's why obese men have breast enlargement and small penises, while obese women have an elevated risk for breast cancer for the same reason.

These fat cells secrete other things, too, including an enzyme known as SCD1. This enzyme, along with TNF, leads to inflammation through the NFkB system.

Treating this with the omega-7 oils alone will decrease it by 73%!

The Cleveland Clinic, in a very short, eight-to-twelve-week study using the Omega-7 oils, found it increased the good cholesterol levels significantly, and decreased the size of plaque in the patient's aorta by 47%. It has also been shown, in other studies, to increase the lining of blood vessel cells through nitric oxide, increasing blood flow. Lastly, the Omega-7 oils have been proven to decrease fatty livers, associated with the metabolic syndrome (early diabetes), and non-alcoholic fatty liver disease, associated with cirrhosis and liver cancer.

You can find the Omega-7 oils in certain foods, like macadamia nuts and sea buckthorn, containing about 20% of the good oils but also 10-40% palmitic acid, negating the good oils by causing clumping of the platelets, arterial stiffness, and raising the LDL levels. Therefore, only use a good supplement not containing these bad guys, *and* avoid these foods.

Here, like in many other examples, the supplements are better than the foods, so don't get stuck in the "all food" mode. Another good illustration is pomegranate, where the supplement is far superior than eating the fruit since it contains extracts from the seeds, fruit, and flowers, and they *all* have separate and unique beneficial chemicals.

Chapter Four

PMS, Menopause, Chronic Fatigue Syndrome, Immunity, and Inflammation

Introduction

Premenstrual syndrome (PMS) and menopause are both hormone related in women, and their changes can have profound physical and mental consequences. Treating them with nutrient therapies can be achieved very nicely and help these women with the day-to-day nightmare. Also, chronic fatigue syndrome is common and pervasive, and many times we find it woven into the landscape of these hormonal problems. I will integrate our immune system into the general discussion and how it relates to it all.

PMS is associated with lower abdominal pain, swelling of the legs and hands, anxiety, insomnia, headaches, muscle aches and cramping just before menstruation (period) begins. Thought to be due to the rearrangement of the hormones (no one knows for sure), the standard medical treatments most times are not very good, but the nutrient ones are. A variant of this, polycystic ovarian disease, can be treated with metformin, a drug used for diabetes, or arginine, AMPK (adenosine monophosphate kinase), and cysteine-glutathione. Take note: primrose, advertised for the same conditions, does not work. With any suggestion of polycystic ovarian disease, the patient should have an MRA X-Ray (MRA is most often used to examine vessels in the brain, neck, kidneys, and legs.) of the brain. These women are susceptible to aneurysms that can rupture spontaneously and cause a cerebral hemorrhage.

More specifically, nutrients include:

<u>Black Cohosh</u>

1. Has four active ingredients and the actions include maintaining and suppressing luteinizing hormone (LH) levels. LH hormone normally is released by the pituitary gland and in turn stimulates production of progesterone from the ovaries.
2. Has an estrogen-like receptor effect, and numerous, randomized, well-controlled studies demonstrated mood elevation. Many times, I use it in combination with flax seed, soy protein, and green tea for PMS, menopause, breast discomfort, excessive bleeding with menstrual periods, or painful periods. It seems to rearrange the hormone levels to where they should be.

<u>Green Tea</u>

The green-tea saga began when it was discovered that people from Southeast Asia lived longer than we did, despite their smoking habits. Then it was reported that Asian women had less breast cancer and Asian men less cancer of the prostrate and heart disease. This led us to conclude that perhaps all the green tea they were drinking and their lifestyle made the difference. The active ingredients are their polyphenols. Their potency is determined by when the leaves are picked. The green and white teas are taken off the trees early, therefore, they have the highest levels of polyphenols; while the teas removed later, like oolong and black teas, undergo oxidation longer, so they have less antioxidants. When buying green tea, read the label. The most active ingredient is EGCG (epigallocatechin gallate) and the one with the most of this is the better brand to buy.

There are other sources of these polyphenols, such as dark chocolate first used by the Aztecs. The ORAC grid, a measurement of antioxidant strength, finds the polyphenols of dark chocolate is ten times stronger than spinach.

1. Its actions decrease the oxidative risk of lipids (hardening of arteries) and heart disease, while increasing nitric oxide and blood flow.
2. With diabetes, it lowers the BSL (blood sugar level), blood pressure, weight, and inflammation.
3. Particularly helpful in patients with reflux issues and peptic ulcer disease. For cancer, a much greater understanding has been achieved. Stated simply, all upper-gastrointestinal tumors from the oral cavity to the pancreas can be positively benefited by using it for treatment and prevention.
4. The University of Minnesota announced green tea decreases tumor genesis by binding the protein growth factor for tumor cells, and interacts with other activating proteins and independent growth factors. Lung-cancer cells are also influenced. Basically, it helps to prevent cancer through cell physiology. Besides upper-gastrointestinal tumors, it has a beneficial effect on preventing and treating breast and prostate cancers.

5. A recent study by Dr. Emily Ho at Oregon State University demonstrated positive benefits of green tea consumption in Lupus patients.
6. Green tea has been shown to decrease inflammation in the brain, grow new neurons called "neurites," and benefit patients with Alzheimer's Disease.

The dose is again brand driven and drinking green will not get you to therapeutic levels unless you drink about four-six cups a day. In addition, don't delude yourself into thinking green tea added to beverages is beneficial.

Indications include: HBP, risk factors for heart disease, diabetes mellitus, upper-gastrointestinal problems — peptic-ulcer disease, reflux — menopause, PMS, chronic fatigue, cancer prevention — especially breast, prostate, upper-gastrointestinal, including pancreas — brain dementias and general medical care. The dose again is brand driven.

Soy

In my estimation, soy is probably one of the most undervalued of all the nutrients.

Soy protein has been shown to have beneficial effects on humans. The Japanese take in about fifty grams a day compared to the USA consumption of one gram a day. You will find soy in other sources like tofu, miso, and tempeh. The chemistry of these chemicals is fascinating but let me make one misconception clear: soy does not cause or make breast cancer worse. The three polyphenols of importance are genistin, daidzem, and equol, which act like estrogen substitutes. They fill the estrogen receptors ahead of estrogen, therefore negating estrogens bad effects.

We now know there are two estrogen receptors, an alpha and a beta. The alpha receptor has been linked to breast, ovarian, endometrial, and colon cancer, but the beta receptors, activated by soy protein, counteract these effects.

1. In a premenopausal woman, soy protein acts like an anti-estrogen, thus blocking the receptors, and in postmenopausal women, it acts like an estrogen exerting its positive influence.
2. It not only regulates the receptors but maintains the relationship of estrone, a weak estrogen, and 16 hydroxyl estradiol, a strong estrogen. In that way, the strong estradiol will not exert its negative influences. The Mayo Clinic did a meta-analysis and found no evidence of soy causing breast cancer.
3. Has been shown to release nitric oxide, improving circulation and blood flow, preventing heart disease, and reducing blood pressure by blocking ACE receptors that cause HBP.
4. Increases the PONS receptor, supporting the good cholesterol in removing plaque from arteries, just like pomegranate.
5. As a good chemical should, soy is also anti-inflammatory; it inhibits NFkB and reduces the expression of the molecule responsible for plaque formation.
6. Soy lowers blood sugar levels by decreasing insulin resistance and assists in utilizing blood sugar.
7. Osteoporosis improves through decreasing inflammatory chemicals and recalcifying bone.

8. Clinical studies have shown it will decrease breast and prostate cancer rates by up to 50% and commensurately decrease the risk of endometrial cancer.

9. The dose is fifteen-to-twenty grams a day with indications of general medical care, PMS, menopause, prevention and treatment of cancer — especially breast, endometrial, and prostate — heart disease, HBP, diabetes, osteoporosis, and, perhaps, inflammation, such as arthritis.

Andrographolide Paniculate

We'll talk about this substance later regarding the treatment of the common cold, but its significance is far more reaching. This Asian herb has bio-components that stimulate multiple points of inflammation. This is very exciting since attacking two points of inflammation is much more effective than one and also eliminates the problem of super infections.

1. Improves genes inhibiting pro-inflammatory compounds, improves inhibition of NFkB, an inflammation linked to calcium and chronic changes.

2. Then, it suppresses genes that suppress TNF and prostaglandin E-2.

It would be indicated for anything inflammatory, acute, or chronic, such as colitis and arthritis, with a recommended dosage of 200 mg a day. Now, we can clinically measure these pro-inflammatories, like TNF and the interleukins. I find it exciting to be able to measure and treat these disease markers with nutrients.

Peony Extract

Of the more recent, exciting discoveries is the anti-inflammatory actions of peony extract. The specifics are more in line with autoimmune diseases — lupus, Sjogren's, scleroderma, polymyositis, etc. Here the patients are making antibodies to their own cells. The extract comes from the white root of the flower, even though the flowers may be of all different colors. The mechanism of action is a turn off of the inflammatory cytokines on the front end and the decreasing of the swelling and redness on the back end.

It can be used for any type of inflammation, but its greatest benefit is in the treatment of arthritis. In the standard practice of medicine for arthritis, I use peony along with the standard anti-inflammatory medications, such as steroids and nonsteroidal analgesics, like Voltaren and Naprosyn, and nutrient add-ons, i.e. mung-bean extract, andrographia, and green-tea extract. By using these combinations, many times, even in severe autoimmune diseases, the stronger, more expensive, and dangerous (carcinogenic) biologicals can be avoided. Chemotherapeutics and the anti-TNF agents are obviously the last resort, but if you can treat any of these conditions with inexpensive, safe nutrients, that's the way to go. I have had several patients with RA where their immune reaction (rheumatoid factor in the blood) disappears with peony and their symptoms disappeared as well.

Peony extract, a plant stretching all the way back to Hippocrates and Chinese/Indian cultures, rebalances our immune systems to put them in harmony.

The indications are for any immune inflammatory problem like Lupus, RA, Psoriasis, Sjogrens, etc. and the dose is brand directed.

Chronic Fatigue Syndrome
It is one the most common disorders seen today and was for a long time considered an emotional problem. But now we know it is secondary to viruses, and could be linked to fibromyalgia; severe muscle aches and pains along with the fatigue. Epstein-Barr and the cytomegalic virus, both herpes viruses, are the main culprits, and can be measured with a simple blood test. Low-grade fevers, swollen neck lymph glands, and repeated infections are its hallmarks. The repeated infections are due to the virus's ability to suppress the immune system, especially the "T" cell line of lymphocytes. It is much more than an isolated, short-term problem because it can lead to lupus, and a blood cancer called lymphoma. More recently, the Cytomegalic virus has been linked to pancreatitis (inflammation of the pancreas). What's interesting is standard medications will not work but nutrient therapies will. Fucoidans, reishi with cistanche, gynostemia pentaphyllum, lipoic acid, zinc, and branched chain amino acids in combination are very effect in suppressing viral replication with an abatement of the fatigue and repeated infections. Just make sure there are no other hidden diseases present that could cause it.

Ginseng

When I first learned ginseng's mechanism of action, as a natural substance that helps the body adapt to stress, exerts a normalizing effect, I said, "Right!" As it turns out, it can help us with both mental and physical stress — in other words, to adapt. The active ingredient is panax, and the more the better. This is where reading the label is so important!

1. Studies have shown ginseng will increase endurance and stamina by sparing carbohydrates and allowing skeletal muscle to oxidize free fatty acids for energy.
2. Releases corticosterone in the adrenal gland; increases memory and learning.
3. Increases immunity in colds, and treats chronic fatigue syndrome.

The dose is very brand-directed. Make sure that the brand you use has the highest amount of panax. The indications include: chronic fatigue syndrome, colds, stress, brain-related problems, general medical care, and helps exercise performance.

Fucoidans

This is a long-chain molecule found in seaweed, studied in the field of glycobiology, and is the main part of the Japanese diet in Okinawa, which may partly explain their extended life span compared to all other societies. Overall, it has been shown to increase tissue regeneration, increase immune function against infections and cancer, and prevents inflammation and cancer mutations.

Specifically, we know:

1. Might bind toxins like dioxin.
2. Improves diabetes mellitus and metabolic syndrome by decreasing insulin resistance.
3. Blocks viruses, particularly the herpes virus, from binding to host cells and replicating

(chronic fatigue viruses). It increases "T" cell activity that kills viruses and tumor cells.

4. Decreases AGEs (advanced glycation end products) while decreasing triglycerides and LDL — the bad cholesterol; good for diabetes and aging.

5. Decreases cell-signaling molecules that generate inflammation called pro-inflammatory cytokines.

The dose is 75-300 mg/day, and the indications include: toxic exposures to such things as dioxins, immune deficiency, chronic fatigue syndrome from the herpes virus, recurrent herpes infections (herpes 1 and 2), arthritis, diabetes mellitus, and metabolic syndrome (early diabetes).

Over the last few years a whole new concept has arisen called "immunosenescense." Meaning, with aging our immune systems get fatigued and don't work the way they should, subjecting us to old diseases, like whooping cough, shingles (herpes zoster), and cancer, we see much more in elderly people. Vaccinations for them are now being recommended in older people, but another strategy would be to "beef up" their "T" cell immunity, which can be done very nicely with nutrients like fucoidan. In fact, this concept, besides fucoidans, can be treated with reishi mushrooms extract and cistanche in combination, which is what I recommend.

To fully understand what I just said, let's review briefly some of the basic immune physiology. The most important cells for virus, fungus, and cancer surveillance are "T" cells, named after the thymus gland that programs them. There are two basic pools of them: 1) "innate" and 2) "adaptive," which function differently but work as a team. The "innate" work immediately, while the "adaptive" must be programed and work later, but the goal is to get rid of the offending agent.

For example, cistanche and an enzymatic activated rice bran chemical can stimulate the innate cells while reishi mushrooms stimulate the adaptive ones. In one study of older mice, within forty-eight hours, it increased these cells five times. The problem is the rice bran enzyme can only be used for three-to-four months, but the others can be used indefinitely. Their clinical indications are rather obvious, but for chronic fatigue syndrome they are very useful adjuncts. In other patients who have a compromised immune system — run down, cancer patients, exaggerated weight loss (anorexia) — they are of great value.

Immunosenescense can also effect the other arm of immunity, the antibody-producing one. Its main function is to eradicate bacteria and help with the "T" cells. What happens here is the antibody attaches itself to the offending agent and then the "T" cell comes along and destroys them both. It's basically a team event! Beta carotene is a good stimulator of these cells, along with bone marrow additives of wheat grass, folic acid, and vitamin B12.

Chapter Five
_____

Grid, Antioxidants, and Longevity

Introduction

Earlier, in "How Mechanism Work," we talked about inflammation, oxidation, and their interplay. But the question is how to practically measure them. In working against oxidation, we have antioxidants. And now, we have a way to measure them.

The ORAC (oxygen radical absorption capacity) grid, mentioned earlier, measures the strengths of antioxidants. The higher the number, the better it is.

We are all made up of atoms comprised of nuclear material surrounded by outer rings full of electrons. If these rings are incomplete, they are unstable and called free radicals. One of the more common is the oxygen free radical seen in nature as rust. Another good example is a sliced apple. Within thirty minutes, it starts turning brown — oxidation.

Antioxidants, on the other hand, can neutralize potential free-radical damage. The recommendation is to consume about 3,000 to 5,000 units of antioxidants daily. But what does that mean?

In truth, 80% of us consume only about 1,000 units per day. To give you an idea how hard-reaching the recommended dose is, the recommended five-a-day fruit and vegetable servings will give you 1,750 units per day. A little short, I would say!

Specific examples will give a better perspective: apples are 218 units, bananas 221, and blueberries 2400 units. God provided us clues in color, drawing us to food sources. Therefore, the deep color of anything we consume should have a sign on it saying, "Eat me." Deep color indicates antioxidants that protect plants and humans, too, when we consume them. They manifest very high levels as measured on the ORAC grid, and partially explain the "French Paradox." The reason is there are other antioxidants in the food they eat and red wine they drink, such as resveratrol and sirtuin that protect them. Vitamin B3 also stimulates these same protein systems where they unwrap acetyl groups off histones in the nucleus of cells to make proteins from the RNA. The highest ratings are found in acai berries, blueberries (bilberries), followed by purple corn. Knowing these facts will now help us understand antioxidants and how to measures its effects.

Pycnogenol

Used in Europe for years, this derivative of a maritime (seaside) pine bark has a dramatic chemistry. The proanthocyanins in it have four clear actions.

1. Stabilizes collagen in joints and other supportive tissue, along with the lining of blood vessels.
2. Increases blood flow, especially with the small blood vessels of the extremities, which is beneficial for the treatment of peripheral neuropathy and numbness in the legs of diabetics

or peripheral vascular disease and pains in the legs with walking from occluded arteries.

3. Has antioxidant activity, including free-radical scavengers.
4. Increases immunity and kills cancer cells.
5. Decreases the pressure in the eye to help treat glaucoma along with bilberry (blueberry).
6. Europeans have used it specifically for venous insufficiency, diabetic neuropathy, HBP, and arthritis. Now, you can add glaucoma. The dosage is, again, brand-directed. Indications include: general medical care, coronary artery disease, peripheral vascular disease, arthritis, glaucoma, diabetes neuropathy, and cancer prevention. The only caveat is it is expensive.

Beta carotene

Beta carotene has gotten a bad rap. The saga really goes back to the early 1980s, when it was found that high-residue foods could prevent colon cancer. Extrapolated from this data was the presumption the beta carotene in these foods was the cause. The beta carotene studies, however, found it did not prevent colon cancer. From that point on, beta carotene became a black sheep in the family of nutrients. This fat-soluble vitamin is found in yellow/orange fruits and vegetables, and is a precursor to vitamin A, also known as carotene. If you overeat it, your skin can turn yellow and is frequently misdiagnosed as jaundice (turning yellow from liver disease).

Beta Carotenes:

1. Increase immunity through the thymus gland, therefore increases "T" cell activity against viruses, fungus, and cancer cells.
2. Support protein synthesis.
3. Are strong antioxidants in protecting DNA.
4. Supportive nutrients to the retina, increasing visual acuity and protecting it.
5. Beta carotene in and by itself does not prevent colon cancer, but it, along with other things from cruciferous vegetables (broccoli, kale, spinach), includes beta isothiocyanate, phloridzin, apigenin, and sulforaphane. Also, mung beans or its extract will do the same thing by creating butyrate that prevents any DNA mutations in the colon.

The standard dosage is, 10,000-25,000 i.u./day. Indications include: visual problems, such as macular degeneration, prevention of colon cancer, chronic fatigue syndrome, to increase immunity, protein-wasting situations with weight loss, and general medical care.

Vitamin B12

1. Vitamin B12 is relatively well-known, but most people do not realize how complicated its absorption is. When consumed, mostly derived from red meats, it requires both stomach acid, secreted by the cells, and intrinsic factor to break down and be absorbed. In this acidic environment, with intrinsic factor attached, it then becomes attached to a pancreatic factor, and finally gets captured by a receptor in the small bowel to be absorbed. If any of these steps are inadequate, the B12 will not be absorbed and a B12 deficiency called pernicious anemia can

develop. Pernicious anemia is precisely what the term means, "wicked low blood." This deficiency can occur with vegetarians since B12 is found in meats, just getting older, or an immune disease causing faulty absorption.

2. Pernicious Anemia manifests as large cell anemia and degeneration of the spinal cord. Long term, it carries a risk of stomach cancer. It takes a long time to develop because we use only about one microgram per day and since the liver stores approximately 5000 mcg, to deplete the liver store house would take about five years.

3. B12 is also intimately involved in DNA metabolism; may be the reason we see an elevated cancer of the stomach in patients with low acid and pernicious anemia.

4. B12 and folic acid are responsible for blood cell maturation in the bone marrow.

Symptoms include: fatigue, tiredness, gait problems, such as a "slapping gait," abdominal pain secondary to gastric ulcer, and cancer. Replacement can be done orally, but it may require under the tongue or monthly injections. B12 levels can be checked with a blood test, along with intrinsic factor and parietal cell antibody tests for confirmation. Incidentally, people who drink too much alcohol can become B12 and folic acid deficient, resulting in a macrocytic anemia, an obvious clue as to their drinking habits. The dose will depend on the degree of deficiency and its progress.

Ashwagandha

An Ayurveda remedy from India, a pepper plant, ashwagandha, is helpful with general metabolism issues and nervous-system problems.

The active ingredient does the following:

1. Decreases oxidative damage to the central nervous system, and regenerates axons and dendrites.
2. Stimulates immunity.
3. Decreases cortisol levels by 26%.
4. Used mostly as a mild tranquilizer, the dose is brand-directed. Indications include: anxiety (especially stress induced), and sleeping problems. Mild and smooth in its action, it can be used with safety. There are no driving restrictions, for example.

DHEA (Dehydroepiandrosterone)

DHEA is a hormone made by the adrenal gland with an interesting history and glowing future. It regulates fat, mineral, and energy function along with decreasing the aging process, including the brain. A precursor to approximately 150 other hormones in the body, it was first discussed in the 1960s by Dr. Vladimir Dillman in his paper, "The Health Project," where he proposed the idea of aging as the result of decrease in natural occurring hormones. His premise was if these hormones, like DHEA, were replaced, the aging process would not occur. It turns out that by the age of twenty-five, DHEA levels peak, but by sixty, the levels have fallen to 40-73% of normal.

Regarding diabetes and the metabolic syndrome (slightly elevated blood sugar, triglycerides, insulin levels):
1. Shifts metabolic balance in favor of usage and not storage of the sugar.

2. Increases insulin sensitivity.
3. Helps to get rid of the free radicals and in the formation of advanced glycation end products (AGE products).
4. Turns off inflammation that may prevent the onset and slow the progression of deadly diabetes, other chronic diseases, and cancer.
5. The decline of our immune systems as we age may also be linked to immunosenescense and a drop in DHEA levels. Replacing the DHEA may obviate this immune deficiency, but studies need to be done. Its antiviral properties may be a clue.
6. The aging process is also a huge factor in mental deterioration and dementia. Studies of elderly people and schizophrenics showed 200 mg/day of DHEA helped both mental and physical problems.
7. Useful in patients with low blood pressure and symptoms of vertigo when they stand.
8. Helps increase bone density in osteoporosis.
9. Counters the immune activity in lupus and has become a primary treatment.
10. Elevates testosterone levels in men for the low "T" syndrome.
11. Helps retina maintain integrity.

The dose will be determined, but corresponding blood levels and indications include: general medical care (aging), immune deficiency and recurrent viral infections, lupus, fatigue, early dementia, diabetes, mental problems, osteoporosis, vertigo, macular degeneration, and, more recently, male sexual dysfunction or low "T" syndrome. Since it converts to sex hormones, like estrogen, both cancer of the breast and prostate need to be considered. One more thing, the DHEA offered at superstores and other wholesale distributers will not work because it is a yam extract, converted to DHEA by an enzyme only found in rats, as I have mentioned previously.

SAM-e (s-adenosylmethionine)

To understand its use, we need to review some brain physiology. Neurotransmitters in the brain are both chemical and electrical, and are interrelated. These chemicals, (serotonin, epinephrine, and dopamine) many times are linked to depression. Their synthesis is dependent on vitamin B12, folic acid, and SAM-e, and while antidepressant medications work on these brain chemicals within the synapse, SAM-e works differently.

1. Affects cell membranes, therefore affecting nerve transmission, along with its ability to activate or suppress specific genes.
2. Affects proteins associated with chromosomes and may prevent certain cancers.
3. The active chemical adds to the synthesis of polyamines and makes cysteine and glutathione for strong antioxidant activity.
4. Has anti-inflammatory properties and can be used to treat arthritis.

The increased phosphatidyl levels in the brain inhibit re-uptake of serotonin and epinephrine, or both, as do antidepressant medications, such as Prozac, Zoloft, Lexapro, etc., while decreasing gamma-aminobutyric acid activity, raising one's mood, and lessening the symptoms of depression.

The dose varies depending on the problem from 50 mg to 1600 mg with the one caveat being its expense. How good is it? A recent study from Harvard reported in the

Journal of Psychiatry that depressed patients who had failed on standard medication but then were treated with SAM-e 800 mg twice daily, showed higher response rates of improvement, up to 105% with remission rates of 121%. Now that is some response.

St. John's Wort

An herbal remedy sometimes called Tipton's weed or chase devil, St. John's Wort is a cure for the common man that has been used for centuries for sadness, worry, anxiety, poor sleep, and depression. It was named after St. John the Baptist because the plants bloom on his birthday (June 24th) and wort is the old English for "plant." The active ingredients are hypericum perforatum and hyperphorin, with many experts stating the latter is the most potent. Twenty studies have shown it to be effective with mild to moderate depression but it takes four to six weeks to experience its full effect, so be patient.

1. Works much like the standard antidepressants work by preventing up-take of serotonin and epinephrine in the brain.
2. Hyperforin also has an affinity for the GABA and Glutamate receptors that also help sedate the brain.
1. Side effects include: light sensitivity in the eyes, dry mouth, and indigestion along with interfering with AIDS drugs and birth-control pills; precautions must be taken. The indications include mild to moderate depression, and the dose is brand-directed. There are many drug interactions, so if the patient is on other medications, I would not use it.

Chapter Six

Nerves and Allergy

Introduction

Nerves, like all cells in our bodies, have a life span and we need to understand their role in your wellbeing, whether it be in the brain or in the peripheral nervous system (arms and legs). Allergic or hyperactive immune systems can affect the whole body.

Neuropathies are diseases of the peripheral nervous system that cause symptoms of numbness of the legs, feet, hands, or all. We see it frequently in diabetics who are poorly controlled. When these symptoms present themselves, your doctor will search for a cause, which most commonly would be diabetes, vitamin B 6 deficiency, Lyme disease, carpal tunnel syndrome, too much alcohol, heavy-metal poisoning, or fish toxicity due to ciguatera poison. Once these problems are investigated, the treatment is directed to them, to the neuropathy itself, or to both. The good news is, in my experience, nutritional therapies are as good as or better than the standard medical therapy, such as Neurontin or Lyrica.

Huperzine

This is a Chinese moss called huperzia serrata. Actions are centered in both the central and peripheral nervous system — the brain, spinal cord, and peripheral nerves. It also promotes healthy vascular tissue in the brain through its immune, metabolic, and antioxidant effect. Several double-blind studies have shown Huperzine to improve the nerves themselves and decrease the numbness of neuropathy.

I use it in conjunction with lipoic acid, vinpocetine, and vitamin B complex with the dose of Huperzine 50 mcg, taken five days out of seven. Be patient. Since the nerves are metabolically inactive, it can take two to three months for it to work. Generally, it slows down the progression first, then improves it.

Vitamin B Complex

Let's discuss the combination of B vitamins.

B1

Also known as thiamine. A deficiency thereof causes beriberi, a condition mostly of historical interest, but sometimes its seen with alcoholics.

B2

Also known as riboflavin, it is directed more toward cell energy production.

B3

Also known as nicotinamide riboside, it stimulates healthy cells, and, subsequently, there is less aging, and cancer mutations. It recently has been linked to sirtuins, along with resveratrol, to remove acetyl groups off histones in the nucleus of our cells that then allow the RNA to make proteins. That is really exciting since it is directly part of the aging process. As we get older, it becomes less effective and, in doing this, we age. It is also related to cellular energy and sugar metabolism that is directly related to diabetes and aging.

Niacin

Niacin has become a major player in the medical profession for treating increased lipids, like triglycerides levels, and lowering Lpa particles (the widow maker), which can cause heart disease. It may cause flushing, redness in the cheeks, and lightheadedness, so it needs to be taken with food.

B6

Also known as pyridoxine, it is associated with neuropathies and INH drug therapy for tuberculosis. A recent study from Taiwan showed it to decrease inflammatory TNF and IL6 markers with RA patients.

Folate

Also known as folic acid, it helps prevent birth defects and heart disease, and stimulates the bone marrow to produce cells in anemic states. When an elevated reticulocyte level in the blood is found, along with anemia and colitis (inflammatory), it is also indicated.

B12

Also known as Cyanocobalamin, it is used to treat pernicious anemia or anemias associated with increased alcohol intake.

<u>Biotin</u>
Works in conjunction with the others.

<u>B5</u>

Also known as pantothenic acid, it works in conjunction
with the others.

Indications for vitamin B complex include: neuropathy,
elevated homocysteine levels (associated with heart
disease), B deficiencies, in pregnancy to prevent birth
defects, colitis, certain dementias, general medical care,
and anemia. Dose, brand-directed. Vitamin B complex
can cause stomach upset; take it with food if possible.
Butterbur

A perennial shrub, this plant is coming into its own. Its
main actions are anti-inflammatory and antispasmodic
of smooth muscle. The active ingredients are isopetasi,
oxopetasis, and petasin, and with their antispasmodic
activity, are important for respiratory function
(preventing constriction of airways) and the constriction
of blood vessels in the brain, the prime cause of
migraines.

1. Isopetasi and petasin inhibit lung inflammatory
    chemicals, while Petasin inhibits COX- 2
    activity, too, therefore reducing inflammation of
    the lungs. COX 1 and 2 drugs are frequently
    used to treat arthritis like Naprosyn, Voltaren,
    and Mobic because they are anti-inflammatories.
2. They also decrease intracellular calcium activity
    resulting in the closure of blood vessels in the
    brain. By opening blood vessels in the brain, the
    headaches improve.

3. Maintains nasal histamine and prevents release, decreasing allergies.

Butterbaur

1. Decreases nausea and vomiting mediated through COX-2 and LOX (Lipoxygenase) enzymes.
2. Many times, you will find butterbur mixed with ginger, riboflavin, and rosemary, with the dose being 75 mg two to three times a day, for migraine headaches and allergy. The allergy indication is also useful for asthmatic patients. Check to make sure it contains no pyrrolizidine. This can cause liver and kidney disease, and present a risk of cancer. It is as good as standard medication for treating allergy, asthma, or migraine headaches, and is cheaper and safer. I once spoke with a neurologist who specialized in headaches and he told me that butterbur was as good as any medications for treating migraines.

Lipoic Acid

A versatile nutrient, it is both water and fat soluble, meaning it can gain access into all cells of the body, including the brain, and fulfills the need for a long-acting antioxidant because of its ability to regenerate glutathione. Glutathione, made in the liver, is made up of three amino acids — cysteine, glutamic acid, and glycine — and is found in the water components of all cells.

1. Regenerates glutathione and neutralizes free radicals to prevent cellular decay.

2. Works in conjunction with acetyl-L-carnitine, preserving mitochondrial function, while protecting the nerves, preventing and/or treating neuropathy, and benefits patients with Parkinsonism and Alzheimer's disease. It not only protects the existing mitochondria that make energy for the cells but grows more called biogenesis. Instead of less and less of them as we age, they grow more.

3. Useful for diabetics, it has an added benefit by improving glucose intolerance along with decreasing obesity, triglycerides, and inflammation of our blood vessels. In doing so, it also decreases our risk of heart attacks and strokes.

4. Increases e NOS (endothelial nitric oxide synthase), that dilates blood vessels and, in turn, increases blood flow.

A new preparation, Na R-Lipoic acid, increases the plasma level by ten to fifty times. It is often taken in conjunction with biotin and vitamin B complex with indications including: heart disease, Alzheimer's, neuropathies, diabetes, muscle disorders, CNS problems, and general medical care with aging. With neuropathies, I use it in combination with vitamin B complex, vinpocetine, and huperzine. For diabetics, I will add pycnogenol for the microvascular component, carnosine, and the omega-3-7 oils. If the target treatments are the mitochondria, I add acetyl-L-carnitine, CoQ10, PQQ, and branched chain amino acids.

<u>Blueberry (Bilberry)</u>

In 1927, in the *Journal of the American Medical Society*, an article appeared stating blueberry is a compound that came close to curing diabetes. Of course, this was before insulin, but the conclusion tells you something. During World War II, they discovered blueberries improved night vision to the extent that Royal Air Force pilots took it routinely for night-time raids. More recently, it has made its presence known on the ORAC grid, where impressively its antioxidant rating was immense. Chemically, blueberries are part of the polyphenol family of chemicals and subfamilies of the flavonoids. The blue color is due to delphinidins that are strong proanthocyanidins.

1. Strong antioxidant action to the point of neutralizing reactive oxygen species (ROS), a very bad, strong free radical. The effects on diabetes are so dramatic, I would recommend all diabetics and metabolic syndrome (or Syndrome X) which is considered prediabetics, patients take it.
2. Helps avoid increased fat tissue, where the sugar we consume goes into fat cells instead of muscles.
3. Slows the absorption of carbs (lowering the glycemic index), while increasing insulin production and insulin sensitivity.
4. Decreases LDL oxidation, thereby decreasing disease of blood vessels in diabetics.
5. Helps prevent cancer by a mechanism that mimics metformin, a medication we use to treat diabetes, improving programmed cell death.
6. Decreases chronic inflammation through blocking inflammatory chemicals, like TNF and cytokines.

7. Maintains cell-signaling pathways that prevent cancer and secures normal cell physiology.
8. Maintains cell reproduction, so cells age gracefully and maintain their function.
9. Neutralizes tumor cell invasion, thus the spreading thereof.
10. Inhibits spread of tumors through blood and lymphatic system.
11. Interrupts the formation of new blood vessels for tumor growth.
12. Protects the retina (a must for diabetics), along with the lens in the eye, and, with pycnogenol, against cataracts. You can see the benefits of decreasing oxidation and the aging of the eye, decreasing permeability of the blood vessels, increasing blood vessel walls and connective tissue strength, preventing leakage of blood or fluid that ages the eye or causes separation of retinal layers leading to blindness.

The dose is again brand-directed with indications including: diabetes, coronary artery disease and its risk factors, visual problems, cancer prevention and treatment, along with general medical care.

The best blueberries are called "aurora blueberries" from Alaska. They contain the highest level of antioxidants. Why? Because to survive in Alaska, the plant truly needs stamina; an expression of its antioxidant levels that you benefit from by consuming them.

Chapter Seven

Lipids and Diet (the "Biggie")

Introduction

The majority of my practice, in general, involves obesity and its dietary management. Many misconceptions and erroneous ideas abound so educate yourself to the *hard* facts.

Obesity is the underlying linchpin for many diseases. From diabetes to heart disease, treatment *always* starts with weight control. Unless you control the weight, success will be extremely unlikely. No matter how many nutrients, medications, or both are used, overweight patients will have poor responses, even if you double or triple the dose and number of medications. In turn, because of physical or mental inactivity, what caused the disease will often increase the obesity — a true negative cycle that needs to be broken.

Obesity is more than just a big belly. These fat storage areas — made up of large fat cells in obese people, as compared to the small, normal ones in non-obese people — are an active endocrine-secreting organ. We also know low carbohydrate diets, such as Adkins and South Beach, are the best at controlling weight over short and long periods. Both maintain good blood parameters, like blood sugar and lipids, because they favor the small fat cells, the good guys. The insulin surge that occurs with carbohydrate ingestion is the main villain, and this surge may also be linked to cancer since insulin is a growth factor. So, let's look closer at some of the physiology.

Obesity can be determined by calculating your BMI (body mass index), a standard measurement we all use now, including your insurance company, but a rather complicated formula. If greater than twenty-five (overweight), then weight needs to be lost. If over thirty, you are considered obese. One caveat: if muscular, you will have a falsely elevated BMI.

All too frequently, we think of obesity as an elevated BMI, bulging waistline, and tight-fitting clothes. That's all true, but the most important thing is the metabolic effect of it on *you*. Those fat cells are not just dormant storage areas but powerhouses for disease and the whole aging process. Let me explain.

There are two types of Adipose cells (fat cells): 1) the small cell, the good ones, and 2) the large cell, the bad ones, as previously mentioned. The small cell secretes a hormone, adiponectin, that decreases fat storage and increases sugar utilization. The large fat cell does the opposite, resulting in insulin resistance and sugar elevation (pre-diabetes, metabolic syndrome, or syndrome X). This cell also secretes TNF, increasing fat storage and inflammation — not good. These larger fat cells also secrete estrogen, a real problem for women with breast-cancer risks, and in men causes breast enlargement and low "T" syndrome (low testosterone), along with shrinkage of their penises.

On the small fat cells is a receptor that helps regulate energy and its transport into the body's cells to lower insulin resistance. Called a "pars" receptor (PPAR,s), it also removes existing plaque and therefore improves what aging has already occurred.

The two receptors have separate activities and, if distinguished, could be targeted depending on what our desired outcome is. One decreases the formation of glucose and the formation of fat cells, along with activating the gene that increases the longevity gene. The second decreases inflammation and increases exercise tolerance. These newly discovered distinct receptors will help target specific problems.

What nutrient can affect these receptors? Pomegranate.

And one word about the liver here, an organ managing many tasks, it digests fats, makes and stores glucose, and serves as the body's detox center. The liver is a warehouse for sugar, stored as glycogen, and if you become sugar deficient, it will be broken down and sugar levels will go up. It also detoxifies many chemicals that could be harmful, such as ammonia. When the liver fails, a person will develop ammonia toxicity. Its functions, of course, decline with age, as everything else does, but there is a tremendous reserve. You can have 80% of your liver removed or destroyed and it will still function normally.

Silymarin aka Milk Thistle

The one nutrient that directly effects the liver and is of great benefit is silymarin, also known as milk thistle.

1. Has a strong antioxidant activity and increases glutathione levels in the liver.
2. Strong anti-inflammatory activity against Cox-1-2, NFkB, and lipo-oxygenase in the liver and throughout the body.

3. Protects patients who are experiencing acetaminophen (Tylenol) overdose.
4. Decreases damage of alcohol on the liver.
5. Protects liver from non-alcohol fatty liver disease.
6. Lowers blood sugar better than diabetic drugs metformin and actos.
7. Protects patients from liver cancer.

Obesity just puts a strain on the liver, as well as on all other organs. It would seem blocking carbohydrates would be a good way to lose weight and promote health. There are two nutritionally basic ways of doing that:

1. L-arabinose inhibitor, a sucrose blocker, prevents blood sugar spikes and only allows 2% carbohydrates to be absorbed.
2. Alpha amylase and glycosidase inhibitors of which there are two: 1) White bean extracts that specifically block complex sugar absorption and increases cholecystokinin (gut hormone-CCK); decreases appetite and triglycerides, and 2) Irvingia.

Irvingia

My favorite, from the wild African mango, it does all the right things.

1. Causes about a 5% weight loss per month along with decreasing lipids and increasing HDL, the good cholesterol.
2. Decreases genes that increase fat production and increases genes that decrease blood sugar.
3. Decreases systolic blood pressure.
4. Increases adiponectin and decreases leptin levels.

5. One study group, on an 1,800-calorie diet, lost 11.5 lbs. as compared to a control group who lost 2.9 lbs. over thirty days. It also seemed to decrease appetite and control metabolic effects. In another study of 120 patients, who took Irvingia 150 mg twice daily for ten weeks, they lost an average of 28 lbs. compared to the control group who lost just 1.5 lbs. Also, body fat decreased 6.3% and the LDL (bad cholesterol) decreased 27% as compared to 1% and 5% respectively in the control group. The dose is 150 mg twice a day with the clear indication being obesity. This nutrient makes sense in decreasing or slowing carbohydrate absorption, not only for weight loss, but improving diabetes and decreasing the cancer risk.

Next are the lipids, a real renaissance in our medical care delivery. Heart disease is the number one killer of Americans, costing us billions of healthcare dollars every year. Before, when we ordered a lipid panel, we had tests for cholesterol, HDL (good cholesterol), LDL (bad cholesterol), triglyceride, and non-HDL, and that was it. Now we know they all can be normal, but you could still be at risk because what's *in them* is *abnormal*. Also, we can now measure other risk factors, like homocysteine levels, Lpa particles also known as the "widow maker," sterols (plant fats that cause heart disease), and even blood omega-3 oil levels. All these micro fractions can be treated independently, which gets you out of harm's way. During your annual physical, insist on these tests! That one blood test not only does blood sugar levels for diabetes but insulin levels and free fatty acids, early indicators of diabetes and metabolic syndrome (syndrome "X") also known as prediabetes.

Meaning, an early diagnosis and treatment of diabetes is mandatory to avoid aging of your blood vessels.

Red Rice Yeast

A red run-off called monascus purpureus is made from the fermentation process over rice. In China, it is regularly used as a preservative, spice, and food coloring seen in Peking duck, fish paste, and red wine. Mevacor, the first cholesterol drug, statin, was derived from it and the Chinese still use it medically for circulation, indigestion, and diarrhea.

1. Monasculins block an enzyme that helps the body make cholesterol in the liver. By inhibiting this enzyme, cholesterol levels go down. And since most of our cholesterol is made in the evening, it is optimal to take it around supper time. All statin medications like Lipitor, Zocor, and Crestor work the same way.
2. A study at UCLA over twelve weeks using red rice yeast showed a significant drop in cholesterol, LDL, and triglycerides but not the HDL, the good cholesterol.
3. Citrinin in it may cause liver toxicity and muscle necrosis, requiring it to be monitored just like all other cholesterol medications with blood tests every three months. If muscle aches and pains occur, stop it immediately. Most times patients with the muscle aches and pains have CoQ10 deficiency and will respond to it. Both statin medications and red yeast rice can do this.
4. Cholesterol levels over 250 and LDL levels over 120 will not respond very well to red yeast rice. The goal for cholesterol to be less than 180 and a LDL under eighty. So, these patents will need

standard medication. The dose is brand-directed and regulated according to the cholesterol and LDL levels.

Indications are those of increased lipid levels and risk factors, such as diabetes, or metabolic syndrome (syndrome X). Frequently, I add guggal, a supplement I will describe in a moment, to increase effectiveness. In my experience, it works as well as the weaker statin medications.

Policosanol

Made from sugar cane, it decreases cholesterol levels.

1. Blocks HMG. Like red rice yeast, binds LDL to degrade it, decreases LDL peroxidase, which forms plaque.
2. Inhibits smooth muscle proliferation, an early stage of atherosclerosis. More recently, arterial stiffness with aging is related to this. In addition, vitamin D3 and K2 w ill reduce this stiffness.
3. Inhibits platelet aggregation, which may help prevent heart attack.

It is very safe, takes three months to work, and is brand-directed regarding dosage, and the dose, of course, will vary depending on the serum cholesterol level. I use this, many times, in tandem with guggal, a blocker of cholesterol absorption from the GI tract after eating. In my experience, it is not quite as strong as red yeast rice, so use it with lower cholesterol levels of 200-220.

Guggal

This Ayurvedic remedy comes from a tree gum resin extract.

The actions include:

1. Blocks cholesterol absorption from the gastrointestinal tract.
2. Decreases lipid oxidation, preventing hardening of the arteries.
3. Increases hepatic sites that bind LDL, decreases cholesterol metabolism, and increases the excretion of bile acids and cholesterol.

On the market, there is a similar drug available called Zetia, part of another drug, Vytorin, containing simvastatin (a statin drug) and Zetia. Sometimes it is included with niacin, with the dose being brand-directed and the clear indication being elevated cholesterol levels. I also use it in conjunction with policosanol or The toxicity is again very low to nonexistent.

<u>CoQ10</u>

It is very hard to categorize since it does a plethora of amazing things. Its main action is with cellular energy production. Chemically, this fat-soluble antioxidant is made in the body, rendering it non-essential.

1. Helps our mitochondria make cellular energy and prevents decay (aging) of them while making new mitochondria, biogenesis. It's done through increasing genes that affect it. In any cell of the body, there may be 2-2,500 mitochondria with different sets of DNAs from the nucleus of the cell and many experts now think the actual number of mitochondria relates to longevity.

Consequently, it is crucial to avoid killers of our mitochondria, such as smoking, drinking too much alcohol, obesity, diabetes, heart disease, and antioxidant overload (free radicals), and all are associated with aging. Since your heart is the most energetic organ of the body, it needs the most energy and is thus most vulnerable.

2. Indirectly affects chemical reactions as a coenzyme, and as an antioxidant is 30-5,000 times stronger than vitamin C. So strong, it neutralizes ROS.

3. Works well with lipoic acid, branched chain amino acids, and carnitine. Do not be surprised to see them combined for the treatment of many heart diseases. More recently, PQQ (pyrroloquinoline quinone) has been shown to work with CoQ10 synergistically and they now are recommended to always to be used together. Easy to remember, CoQ10-PQQ.

Indications include: any heart or muscle disorder including hypertension, along with Parkinsonism. Also, anyone taking a statin medication for cholesterol should be on it because the statin medication causes a loss of it in the cell, a culprit of muscle aches and pains. Any form of heart disease, as mentioned, congestive heart failure, coronary artery disease, and arrhythmias (abnormal heart rhythms). The dose can vary considerably from 200-1000 mg/day, along with PQQ. Go by your doctor's recommendation after evaluating your history and what you are taking now. It should be considered as part of your general medical care and anti-aging strategy.

PQQ

PQQ (Pyrroloquinoline Quinone), synergistically works with CoQ10 on many of these effects. Look for a combination of the two when possible.

1. Neutralizes ROS with its antioxidant effect.
2. Protects against tissue being cut off during a stroke and decreases the size of stroke injury.
3. Helps remove mercury in the brain.

For cardiovascular systems:

1. Activates signal proteins in the heart; the heart cells function better and live longer.
2. Activates the gene that decreases blood pressure, cholesterol, and triglycerides.
3. Protects DNA.
4. Protects us from cell death.
5. Probably the most common indication for their use is taking statin medication for an elevated cholesterol level. All statin medications — Lipitor, Crestor, etc. — deplete PQQ/CoQ10 and is part of the reason people get muscle fatigue while taking it.
6. Last, but not least, it sometimes has dramatic anti-cancer affects, particularly with breast and colon cancer. It blocks new blood-vessel growth that allows tumors to grow and spread.

Clinical studies to date show heart attack rates can decrease from 45% to 25% with a dose of 120 mg/day. Breast and colon cancers decreased by 25-53% at the same dose range. The dose can vary for CoQ10 from 120 mg/day to 1,200 mg and PQQ 20 mg/day. In fact, when treating or preventing Parkinsonism, a dose of 900-1,200 mg/day of the CoQ10 is recommended. Also, because of their symbiotic actions, selenium, vitamins E and C and EPA oils may be added.

Indications include: Parkinsonism, congestive heart failure, HBP and risk factors for heart disease, statin medication, cancer prevention, muscle problems including chronic fatigue, fibromyalgia, and general medical care. Look for ubiquinol because its absorption is far superior to ubiquinone with added PQQ and lipoic acid. If you had to pick one nutrient to take, CoQ10/PQQ would be a good one.

Chapter Eight

Joints, HBP (Hypertension), and Vitamin K2

Introduction

These two areas have new research updates and understandings well served by nutrient therapies. Some will surprise you. They did me. For example, Vitamin K2 is a great clinical add-on with new insights.

Glucosamine

A natural occurring amino acid, it is made up of glucose and L glutamine, which decreases with age and have no real food source. Commercial shell fish is the source of most of these supplements, so be careful if you have an iodine allergy. Research tells us that a sulfate group, like glucosamine sulfate, may be more effective, so seek this in the brand you buy. It may also help contribute to cartilage growth component.

Glucosamine improves joint function by two mechanisms:

1. Lubricant. N acetyl glucosamine and glucuronic acid are reconfigured to hyaluronic acid, a joint lubricant (you will find this concentrated chemical in rooster's comb, now standardized into a drug injected into joints to oil them called Hyalgan).

2. Helps stimulate production of glycosaminoglycans, enabling cells to hold together. Studies have shown not only clinical improvement but an increase in joint cartilage growth. But it takes about three months to start working. Patience is the key.

The dose must be at least 1,500 mg/day. Read the label to ensure the only indication is osteoarthritis. I use it in conjunction with MSM and chondroitin, with the latter decreasing joint inflammation. It's used mostly for osteoarthritis (wear and tear), not the immune arthritis's like RA or lupus, and mostly of the knees and hands. Useful add-ons include: mung bean extract, Zyflamend, curcumin, and un-denatured collagen. It goes without saying that if overweight, treatment also includes weight loss, which is *vitally* important. Otherwise it's like treating asthma and the patient continues to smoke.

MSM (methylsulphonylmethane)

A sulfur donor, its significance becomes apparent when we realize sulfur ranks third in body substance and decreases with age.

1. Helps increase immunity of the knee, and supports joint function by donating sulfur groups for cartilage.
2. Decreases joint inflammation and degeneration.
3. Remember, sulfur is critical for amino-acid usage in the repair of cells no matter where in the body, so it should help elsewhere. The dose is brand-directed and used in conjunction with glucosamine for osteoarthritis, tendinitis, along with the other recommendations (see above).

This is very 'handy' for soft tissue joint problems like bursitis and tendinitis.

Un-denatured Collagen

Fifty-two million people in the United States suffer from arthritis. The two major ones, rheumatoid arthritis (RA) and osteoarthritis, were thought to be due to an immune reaction to the joint linings, and wear and tear over time, respectively.

Stanford University was the first to suggest this was not true and that both conditions are based on the same pathophysiology. Researchers found that regardless of the initiator mechanism (wear and tear or immune antibodies), the basic underlying origin in both resulted from the exposure of joint collagen. Yes, two very different conditions — an immune reaction or wear and tear — caused by the same basic problem. This exposure of collagen causes "T" cells to be activated, resulting in the inflammatory reaction previously mentioned. These killer cells start the inflammatory-chemicals cascade with resulting arthritis. Arthritis causes terrible problems — patients can't walk, gain weight, and develop diabetes, hypertension, and heart disease — a truly negative cycle where patients become basically incarcerated in their own bodies. It hurts to move, so they don't move.

"Oh, it's just arthritis." I hear this all the time, but these people are truly suffering. Worse, they become immobile, gain weight, and develop diabetes and heart disease, driving up health-care costs for all of us, all of which is avoidable. Standard arthritis medications work well, but they are expensive, have many side effects, and still do not treat the root problem. So, what can we do to treat arthritis problems at their root cause?

Knowing it is an allergic condition, researchers felt, perhaps, a "reverse vaccination" would be the way to go. We have used this technique for years in patients who have standard allergies, such as hay fever. They come in for their injections of the allergens at low doses that are gradually increased over time. The theory of oral toleration is the body will develop blocking antibodies gradually or "immune fatigue," and the allergies will improve.

The next step was to find a joint collagen product. It turns out chicken cartilage is almost identical to human collagen, so that's what was used. "T" cells employed by joints are programed in the peyer patches, located in the small intestine, which determined the desensitization process had to be oral. Also, the collagen had to have the same molecular, three-dimensional shape (stoichiometric) of human cartilage, requiring the chicken collagen be un-denatured (not unwrapped). You see, when you cook something, the molecules unwrap, destroying its use. Therefore, the chicken cartilage had to be uncooked. This is a step researchers avoided at Harvard by giving patients un-denatured (not cooked) cartilage orally, from chickens. In patients with RA. they found, after three months, there was a significant decrease in joint pain and swelling, and 14% went into complete remission. Beyond amazing! It is spectacular because RA is much harder to treat than osteoarthritis, and just using a nutritional supplement with these results is hard to believe.

Later, a much larger study was done on juvenile rheumatoid (Still's disease) patients with similar results. There have also been other studies of patients with osteoarthritis with similar results spaced out over ninety days. In a head-to-head study, using the un-denatured collagen vs glucosamine over ninety days, the collagen had a reduction of arthritis symptoms by 33% and glucosamine 14%. But the glucosamine in the study was in a sub dose amount and did not include MSM or chondroitin, and my treatments would include *all* of them.

For rheumatoid and osteoarthritis, consider un-denatured collagen as a basis for therapy, in conjunction with mung bean extract, peony extract, curcumin (anti-inflammatory), and glucosamine (1500 mg/day) for osteoarthritis with chondroitin and MSM added.

In my experience, despite their effectiveness, standard medications may be necessary in the more severe cases. You don't want to refuse to take them if your doctor thinks it's best. Remember, chronic inflammation, even in our joints, has long-term consequences for not only the joints but the whole body. These free radicles will affect other organs through the blood stream. In addition, the chronicity will result in scarring and more joint destruction, leading to long-term disability and even surgery. In my arthritic patients, especially with the chronic ones, physical therapy can be a great help to decrease symptoms by increasing joint mobility and preempting joint destructions with deformity. Don't let the innocuous nature of arthritis underplay treatment. Usage of over-the-counter Advil or Aleve for pain relief is a presumption for long-term disaster. Let's not forget arthritis, with inactivity, leads to bigger, devastating but all-preventable problems, like diabetes, cancer, and heart disease. My strategy is to be aggressive with arthritis (front end) and hopefully pre-empt diabetes and heart disease (back end), and, in the process, enhance your quality of life.

Ginger

Ginger comes from a root as a volatile oil named zingiber officinale. As a food additive, it has been around for a long time in such things as ginger beer soda and ginger cookies.

1. Increases prostaglandin E2, a Cox-2 derivative, along with decreasing inflammatory chemicals.
2. Affects Thromboxane B by decreasing it, a Cox-1 system, resulting in a significant decrease in inflammation.
3. Induces programmed cell death in leukemia and colon cancer cells.
4. Stimulates digestive enzymes and increases the secretion of bile, decreasing nausea and vomiting. The dose is 500 mg three times a day with indications of preventing cancer, leukemia, nausea, vomiting, motion sickness, and arthritis. The main use is gastrointestinal and arthritis. If you have a child who gets car sick, or you're going on a cruise, knowing you have had motion sickness before, consider eating ginger snap cookies or drinking ginger beer soda twenty-four hours before you leave or take the supplement. For adults, ginger has made a resurgence comeback with the alcohol drink, Moscow Mules (ginger beer and vodka). I drink it for medicinal purposes, of course.

Hawthorne

A Native American and European plant, it has been used since the Middle Ages. It has three clinical uses:

1. Congestive Heart Failure. An analysis of eight clinical studies showed shortness of breath decreased and exercise capacity increased, all hallmark symptoms of this illness. Hawthorne, carnitine, lipoic acid, CoQ10/PQQ, acetyl-L-carnitine, and branched chain amino acids are a great cocktail for supporting the heart muscle mitochondria.

2. HBP (Hypertension also known as High Blood Pressure). Through ACE inhibition, which causes hypertension, in combination with CoQ10/PQQ/omega-3 oils, it is very effective in lowering blood pressure in the range of 160/100. In my experience, blood pressures over this, especially the second or diastolic reading, are more difficult to treat and generally require standard medication.

3. Arrhythmia (abnormal rhythms). May benefit with fast heart rates like atrial fibrillation. Taurine, an amino acid that decreases sympathetic input, and magnesium may also help along with EPA oils, CoQ10 to reduce and/or convert the arrhythmia.

In summary, its actions are to increase the heart's contractions, ACE inhibition, improvement of heart muscle mitochondria, and a decrease of peripheral resistance with the dose of Hawthorne being brand-directed, generally given twice a day. In my experience, it works, but only on the lower end of hypertension. You will run into complications if you use it for higher levels.

Vitamin K2

The medical profession views vitamin K as an integral part of our body's clotting mechanism. If we did not have the innate (natural) ability to spontaneously clot, we would all bleed to death. The reason why is that internally our blood vessels have pressure points that do micro rupture every day, but this clotting mechanism, through vitamin K, immediately stops the bleeding.

There are two mechanisms, both vitamin K dependent, available to us: the "intrinsic" and "extrinsic" systems. The intrinsic mechanism concerns itself with internal bleeding, while the extrinsic one has to do with external bleeding through the skin or GI tract. Vitamin K1 is responsible for both mechanisms. If you are deficient in vitamin K1, which is made in the liver, you could have a serious bleeding problem. Coumadin, a drug we use frequently as an anticoagulant, inhibits vitamin K1; its main objective.

Now we know there are three types of vitamin K, labeled vitamin K1, K2, and K3, and come from different food sources. K1 is found in green leafy vegetables. K2 is found in dairy, egg yolks, organic meats, and soy. K3 is still under study. Note: 25% of vitamin K comes from our diet, while 75% comes from the bacterial flora in our small intestine, which explains the bleeding problems seen with people on long-term antibiotics that kill the bacterial flora. Another important mechanism of action with vitamin K2 has to do with its relationship to calcium with bone and blood vessels by moving calcium from the arteries to bone.

1. It does so through three chemicals that allow calcium to go from blood vessels to bone, a good thing. If K2 is deficient, the opposite occurs where calcium goes from bone to blood vessel;

the harbinger of atherosclerosis. Therefore, vitamin K2 is also a regulator of calcium mechanics.

2. Many published studies reference vitamin K2, but they all generally focus on its anti-cancer, fracture, and heart effects. A Japanese study looked at vitamin K2 pertaining to fracture rates and found it decreased them by 52%.

3. The Mayo Clinic, in the *Journal of Cancer*, reported a decreased risk of non-Hodgkin's lymphoma, while a small study of forty women found K2 decreased liver cancer rates in patients with cirrhosis by five-fold.

4. Cellular studies showed it decreased growth and invasion of liver-cancer cells, while freezing cell cycle and blocking replication. The vitamin also beneficially affected leukemic, brain, colon, stomach, and prostate tumors.

5. An interesting observation involves the "Triage Theory." It's believed that with stress, vitamin K2 is shuffled over to the coagulation side because of its immediate, survival function, exposing its cancer-prevention action. There may be some relevancy here, making supplementation very rational.

6. Inhibits accelerated growth of cancer cells. Sugar is not allowed to go into the cancer cells to help them grow.

7. Vitamin K2 has been shown to decrease new blood vessel formation for tumors to grow and, with vitamin K3, for DNA-building enzymes.

8. A Rotterdam study of 4,800 patients, over seven to ten years, demonstrated a decrease in heart disease by 57%, with patients having the top one-third vitamin K2 levels.

9. With aging and lower levels of vitamin K2, we see osteoporosis and arteriosclerosis where calcium has shifted from bone to blood vessels.

Presumptive proof is seen in patients who take coumadin over a long period of time, a drug that inhibits vitamin K2. They develop osteoporosis and accelerated heart disease as a result. This means people on long-term coumadin need to be mindful of this and take the necessary precautions, such as a yearly DEXA scan (for osteoporosis) and monitoring of cardiovascular risk factors every year. Recently, rats, genetically bred to lack the protein that uses K2, developed accelerated calcium in their blood vessels and died within weeks of heart disease.

The dose of vitamin K2 is generally 50 mg/day and is brand-directed. Indications include: general medical care, heart disease, atherosclerosis, leukemia, osteoporosis, cancer, and liver disease. People with advanced blood-vessel disease, like carotid disease, are excellent candidates for K2 since it will not only prevent new plaque but remove existing plaque. I use it in this scenario with EPA oils and pomegranate.

Chapter Nine

Food, Pauling, and Sleep

Introduction

All three of these are related, and in medicine, too.

Food

Food can have profound medical consequences. Our diet is loaded with carbohydrates, fats, sugars, and omega-6 oils — all bad! If you are obese, a BMI (body mass index) greater than thirty, then you need to lose weight, but do it in a safe and healthy way. Here, again, I recommend to my patients the Adkin's diet, advocating a restriction of carbohydrates. The results are weight loss, a loss of appetite, and an improvement in blood panels, i.e., cholesterol, blood sugar, etc. If the patient is barely overweight, BMI twenty-five to twenty-nine, then I recommend the Mediterranean diet. This will help them lose weight and maintain healthy blood lipid and sugar levels, too, but it is much more gradual. In the Mediterranean countries, you see very little obesity, and this is a major reason why. Carbohydrates lead to insulin surges, which are linked to obesity, inflammation, and cancer.

Being a vegetarian does not necessarily bestow on you a prolonged, disease-free life but it can end up making you deficient in certain nutrients like vitamin B12, folic acid, conjugated linoleic acid, carnosine, carnitine, vitamin D, and calcium, just to name a few.

Vitamin C

Vitamin C, or ascorbic acid, is a water-soluble vitamin found not only in fruit but in green leafy vegetables. Dr. Linus Pauling made it famous with his outrageous advice to take thousands of milligrams per day when the RDA (recommended daily allowance) is 75 mg to prevent and treat infections by increasing immunity! Years later, it was found that Pauling was right and they (the experts at the time) are still wrong; a finding that doesn't entirely surprise me since he won two Nobel Prizes in biochemistry. Vitamin C deficiency can lead to scurvy (a blood and blood vessel disease); the main reason why the English are sometimes referred to as "limeys" even today. They realized hundreds of years ago that by eating vitamin C rich limes every day while at sea, they would not get scurvy. They did not know why, but it worked.

Vitamin C has been found to increase immunity by:

1. Increasing antioxidant effect.
2. Increasing the WBC count.
3. Increasing interferon and antibodies, "B" cells mediated against bacteria.
4. Increasing "T" cell mediated response against viruses, fungus, and cancer.
5. Increases the absorption of iron and helps convert folic acid to its active form.
6. Decreases histamine release (antihistamine) and is necessary for steroid and carnitine synthesis, meaning it is good for stress-related problems and allergies.

7. Maintains vascular capillary fragility seen in older people with the bleeding into the skin after trivial trauma. Grape seed extract does the same, and they work together great.
8. Do not buy the fancy brands since they are no better and only cost more than the standard vitamin C. The dose for men is 3,000 mg/day and for women 2,000 mg/day with indications including: general medical care, allergies, decreased immunity with repeated infections, prolonged stress, capillary bleeding problems, especially into the skin, and it might help in iron deficiency.

If I feel a cold coming on, I take 3,000 mg of vitamin C daily with ginseng. And guess what? No cold! I know this is anecdote and not hardly a study, but the facts are the facts. Only kidding, just an observation.

The Common Cold

The common cold can be caused by approximately 150 different viruses. That's why we cannot get vaccinated for the common cold. Since they are viruses, antibiotics will not work, which leaves us with treating the symptoms, such as a fever, runny nose, or sore throat. On the bright side, there are natural remedies that can help.

Echinacea

Everyone has heard of Echinacea, but does it work? A meta-analysis of fourteen studies, meaning a review of smaller studies with conclusions derived, revealed cold symptoms were decreased by one to five days. Also, the University of Connecticut discovered Echinacea prevented colds by 58%. Andrographis paniculata in (Kold Kare), according to American and Canadian researchers, improved cold symptoms by 55%. In addition, Cold-FX with ginseng, according to Health Canada (their FDA), will decrease frequency, severity, and duration of colds, and can also be found with standardized ginseng or panax. As an added benefit with this remedy, you can take it long term, two daily as a prevention.

Zinc

Zinc has been advertised for years as a cold remedy and it turns out it does work. Studies have shown it decreases cold symptoms by four days, cough by one-point-five days, and runny nose by one-point-five days. More importantly, inflammation blood markers decrease; an indication it is working metabolically.

Zinc also helps with influenza because it prevents the virus from attaching to the lung lining. It also prevents replication, a direct link to how strong it is. Be careful with zinc. If you use more than 50 mg/day, you can develop a copper deficiency, for which I would recommend copper supplements.

Vitamins C and D

Dr. Linus Pauling advocated vitamin C in high doses, 2000 mg/day women-3000 mg/d men, for the prevention and treatment for colds. Also, in the *Journal of Nutrition*, vitamin D3 (200 i.u./day) decreased cold and flu symptoms by 40%. The normal dose of vitamin D is 5,000 i.u./day, which we recommend for general maintenance to prevent cancer.

In summary, you can see we can deal with the common cold symptomatically, but not really eradicate the virus by using nutritional means. To prevent colds, it seems only ginseng, zinc, vitamin C, and Echinacea work. Now, if someone is sick with a cold or is experiencing cold/flu season, you know what to do.

Now, back to obesity.

Hoodia

Patients, because of their frenzy to find the easy way out of obesity, will grasp for the most ridiculous things. Hoodia is one of them. I mention it only to advise you *not to use it*. From Africa, there are no real studies showing it works and there may be a problem with it causing kidney disease. The supposition was that since most people from Africa are skinny, it must be due to something that they are consuming, like Hoodia. Hoodia, however, *does not* cause weight loss, but the lack of food in Africa does!

Nutraceuticals, Stanols, Sterols

Because something is branded "nutraceutical" (food with medical benefit), it does not mean organic or it has any medical benefit. Rather, these are foods having a medical advantage when consumed.

Nutraceuticals are, for the most part, derived from a plant's soluble fiber, which targets cholesterol in the form of stanols and sterols. Stanol is better because it is absorbed more efficiently and stays in the body longer (up to three months). Some examples would include: Benecol, a Stanol from a pine tree, orange juice with sterols, and eggs fortified with EPA oils. Two grams per day will decrease LDL levels from 6-17%, but don't take sterol or stanol pills. They do not work.

Olive oil is a nutraceutical, too, as we have discussed, but there are more. Brandeis University created a butter-like substance years ago called Smart Butter, a clear example of one. You will also find them in candy bars, milk, chickens, eggs, and cereals.

There will be many more nutraceuticals coming, so remember the basics and don't be fooled. In my opinion, the EPA eggs are much better for you than standard ones.

Sleep and rest, and the lack of them have been more and more in the news. We now know sleep deprivation causes everything from weight gain to heart disease so let's talk about some ways to combat that.

Valerian

Valerian was first described as useful for sleep by two ancient Greeks, first Hippocrates and then Dioscorides in his *De Materia Medica* treatise. Then along came Galen around 100-200 A.D., who called it "Phu" because it smelled so bad, but also recommended its usefulness for sleep.

Controlled studies have shown valerian to work for insomnia and to be as good as valium with no withdrawal symptoms or addiction problems. It may take up to fourteen days to work and rarely does one dose work. Patience, again, is crucial. Remember, it really does smell bad! The dose is brand determined.

1. Kava

A South Pacific dried rhizome (root), kava has been used for centuries in ceremonial proceedings and a welcome drink. Binds to GABA receptors to calm you down, decreases the uptake of stress hormones, and relaxes muscles while not affecting brain function.

2. Decreases anxiety without developing tolerance. Many sleeping pills and tranquilizes have this effect, meaning, with chronic use, they will become ineffective unless you increase the dose, a precursor for addiction, tachyphylaxis. Indications include: anxiety and insomnia. The dose is brand-directed. Liver toxicity has been reported, so liver tests need to be monitored every three months.

Melatonin

Made in the nucleus of the hypothalamus in the brain, it is transferred to the pineal gland for storage and released at night, when it is dark, to initiate sleep. It uses a receptor system (ball in a mitt) in the brain to work, and that's why it's considered a hormone. For those reasons, the bedroom needs to be dark when you go to sleep. So, turn off the TV, phone, and any other light source. Also, e-books give off a blue light that does the same thing; interferes with your sleep. If you want to read at bedtime, use a regular book. We know levels decrease with age and may be responsible for jet lag and other issues related to working night shifts.

1. Involved with new blood vessel formation, especially important concerning cancer.
2. Increases immune response (kills cancer cells) and helps with free-radical removal (inflammation).

3. New data, surprisingly, has revealed night-shift workers, who have decreased melatonin levels, incur an accelerated cancer risk, especially of the colon, breast, prostate, and lung.

Indications include: insomnia, jet lag, and the prevention of cancer for night workers. I recommend night workers take a melatonin supplement when they get home, during the day, before they go to sleep, to help with this. The dose is 20 mg. It is interesting to note the drug Rozerem, used for insomnia, works by using the same melatonin receptors. I tell my patients it will work great or not at all. There is no in between.

Lavender

An aromatic shrub, it is commonly found in Europe and North America. It has volatile oils in it with four active ingredients:

1) Coumadin
2) Phytosterols (plant hormones)
3) Flavonoids
4) Triterpenes

Historically, it has been used by Arabs, Greeks, and the Romans. In fact, the Latin word for wash is *lavare*. Ancient Persians used it as a disinfectant; the Tibetan monks and Buddhists for psychiatric purposes. From an Ayurvedic standpoint, it was used for depression and digestion.

1. Has antispasmodic and antidepressant properties, which makes sense, but its greatest benefit is relaxation.

2. A German study showed some usefulness with sleep and stomach-related problems.

The dose is brand-directed. Indications include: anxiety, sleep problems, and stomach pain/upset. At times, yoga instructors will use it at the end of a session to totally relax. I've tried it, it works, and it smells good, too. Then there is folklore from France that says lavender's fragrance will keep scorpions away, so they put it in their window boxes. If you live in an area where they reside, keep it fresh and sprinkled around your rooms. Just as an aside, Europeans will put geraniums in their window boxes, not as a decoration, but to keep mosquitoes away as they don't like the smell.

Chapter Ten

Eyes, Bladder, Stomach, Pregnenolone, Probiotics, and Garlic

Introduction

Our eyes, many times, take a back seat to other health concerns. But eye disease, for the most part, is preventable, and knowledge is priceless protection. On the same note, stomach and urinary track/bladder disorders are very common, mostly because of our lifestyles.

I will outline how nutrients improve these, and the "Do No Harm" mantra of every medical practice.

Lutein, Zeaxanthin, Blueberries, and Others

We've already discussed macular degeneration, the most common cause of blindness in the USA every year. It can occur in only one eye with the initial systems being very subtle, gradual, and unnoticed until it is too late. That's why a routine yearly eye exam is imperative!

There is nothing worse than to suffer the consequences from a disease that could have been prevented. The nutrient approach is inexpensive and effective, but standard medical treatments may be necessary as well. In addition, no reason exists why they can't be used in tandem. In that case, less of the more expensive medications would probably be a good idea. I can't stress it enough, an early diagnosis and early treatment will prevent blindness!

You know from God's creation clues, the retina is very color dependent. Therefore, foods or related antioxidants with bright colors are necessary to prevent retinal diseases and treat them. Blueberries (bilberries), carotene, lutein, and zeaxanthin are a good start. Add zinc, CoQ10, and glutathione for further antioxidant support, along with resveratrol to help prevent vascular endothelial growth factor in macular degeneration, which, by the way, is what the expensive eye injections are for. More recently, camosine, bilberries, pycnogenol, or maritime bark are being used to prevent cataracts. Lastly, maqui berry extract is being used for dry eyes, but takes about four weeks to work, so again, be patient. Those are my recommendations.

As I mentioned before, during World War II, English pilots ate blueberries (bilberries) prior to flying because it improved their night vision, therefore allowing them to shoot down German planes during night raids. I can't emphasize how important it is to protect your eyes, especially those people with fair complexions with blue or green eyes, who tend to have more issues as they get older. Although those with darker complexions and brown eyes still may have problems, scientific research shows they incur fewer instances.

Cranberry

Wonderful at Thanksgiving, but it is great year-round for treating UTIs (urinary tract infections). Medically, it has been used for over a hundred years, but because of some of its caveats, often not used correctly. In addition to UTIs, stomach ulcers can be benefited also. Preventing and treating stomach ulcers and bladder infections are mediated through three mechanisms:

1. Acidifies the urine, inhibiting bacterial growth and decreasing their swimming ability.
2. Provides strong antioxidant activity.
3. Prevents the bacteria from adhering to the bladder wall to prevent infection. Decreases the binding force twelve times, using what's called a "FIM" mechanism on the receptor site. Remember, it must be taken every twelve hours, otherwise the bacteria already there will adhere and cause an infection. Don't miss one dose!
4. Decreases H. pylori (the bacteria that causes ulcers and cancer of the stomach) growth in stomachs from 14% to 5%.

Indication is recurrent bladder infections. Must be taken for two years for the prevention of gastric cancer and ulcer disease. The dose is brand-related.

Here's a thought, with stomach disorders, try DGL (Deglycyrrhizinated licorice) and cranberry extract. Cranberry Juice will help, but it is loaded with calories and sugar, making the supplements the best way to go. CranActin is better since it contains no sugar, is calorie free, in pill form and is highly concentrated. Again, an ounce of prevention is worth a pound of cure.

Lastly, licorice (the American type, not English) prevents bacterial attachment and accelerates healing by increasing mucous protection. The English licorice can cause hypertension. More recently, zinc has been shown to decrease stomach inflammation and inhibit the H.

pylori bacteria also. I have used it on my patients and found it very effective.

Parenthetically about bacteria... When you study bacteria and how dangerous certain bacteria are, consider these things. Does it produce toxins or have antibiotic resistance? Does it spread easily? Is it "sticky?" Sticky bacteria are more dangerous because they can stick to human tissue, allowing them to grow and result in infections. Cranberry prevents that "sticky" mechanism along with slowing down their motility. A study done at the Brigham and Women's Hospital in Boston of 150 patients showed it does indeed prevent infections.

Indications include: treating and preventing urinary tract infections, more specifically bladder infections. The dosage is 500 mg every twelve hours.

Very recent studies also tell us using probiotics will also help you prevent recurrent infections by keeping the "bad" bacteria under control by about 30%. Meaning, use of probiotics and cranberry extract together is optimal, which is what I do.

Chromium

This is one of the few examples of a trace element that can be used as a single agent for treatment. Chromium normally decreases with age and plays an integral role in diabetes. It improves diabetic blood sugar control and, in turn, decreases infections.

1. Helps lower blood sugars by decreasing insulin resistance, along with supporting glucose tolerance and utilization.

2. May improve cardiovascular function and assist in weight loss. Clinical studies from Georgetown University reported chromium supported lean muscle mass and helped lower blood sugar. The dose is brand-determined with diabetes its main indication. Heart disease, weight loss, and muscular disease are weak secondary indications. One last thing, I would *not* recommend women buy the picolinate type since there may be a risk of ovarian cancer.

Vitamin E

Probably the most important action of vitamin E is its antioxidant effect. There is a lot of misinformation about it, such as it can cause bleeding, not true. Also, you may hear of dosage misconceptions of which I will explain later.

It comes in two forms: a powder, which is readily absorbed, and an oil-based product, which is much easier for most people, including yours truly, to take. But if you're a purist, take the powder.

1. Scavenges the free radicals of lipids, and is also the first defense against lipid peroxidase, therefore a 'chain breaking' antioxidant.
2. Increases immunity against certain cancers, such as prostate and breast.
3. Increases cognition and protects the eyes.
4. Increases cardiac cellular metabolism.
5. Initiates programmed cell death within the DNA proteins, assisting in cancer prevention.

Sometimes vitamin E is combined with selenium; look for the combination. One word of advice, don't take it with vitamin C. They don't get along, so allow a two-hour buffer when taking vitamin C.

Of all the vitamins, vitamin E, or tocopherol, needs to be natural because the synthetic is poorly absorbed. Here, especially, you need to read the label to find out which one is natural and which one is synthetic. You also need to know there are eight isomers, with the most important being alpha and gamma, that need to be in the product and on the label. The label needs to read 'alpha and gamma d tocopherol' not 'alpha dl tocopherol,' the synthetic. The key is the letter "l".

Indications include: eye problems, cancer, CNS (Central Nervous System), and cardiac problems including hyperlipidemia, immunity, and general medical care. The dose is 400-800 µg/day. As an addendum, just recently Tocotriene Ultra, a super-duper vitamin E, has been released that dramatically reduces triglycerides by 30-40%. Add it to your list, with a dose of 250 mg/day.

Last, but not least, for the metabolic syndrome or syndrome "X" (early diabetes) it has become a great adjunct, just like the omega-7 oils. Early diabetes or pre-diabetes is characterized as an elevated blood sugar, with a fasting blood sugar between 100-150 and triglyceride level of over 150; a risk factor for heart disease.

Grape Seed Extract

It is most interesting how many health-oriented organic shoppers don't know how to shop for grapes. It sounds trivial, but believe me, it is on my list of "biggies." We know that dark grapes, ones marked "eat me," contain proanthocyanidins, saponins, resveratrol, sirtuins, and other things that keep the French alive — French Paradox — and will keep us alive, too, if we would only consume them. Not the light green grapes. As an extension of this, why even drink white wine when you can drink red wine and receive seven times more benefit?

When buying grapes, get the ones with the seeds in them because the seeds contain concentrates of the good guys. Grapes with the seeds, or the nutritional-supplement grape seed extract, are also called prebiotics and help our gut flora grow good bacteria (probiotics), our soldiers who protect us from bad bacteria and provide vitamin K and folic acid.

In addition:

1. Rapidly absorbs free radicals and supports the metabolism of collagen in hair, skin, and nails.
2. Protects our CNS by neutralizing ROS — strong free radicals — in our brains.
3. Decreases capillary fragility, mainly in our skin, and prevents bleeding into it.

Indications include: brittle nails, hair problems, such as alopecia (hair loss), along with protecting our brains and bruising on the skin. Common sense also tells us its strong antioxidant activity would benefit many other things yet to be found. The dose is 100 mg twice a day and supplement that by eating red grapes every day with seeds in them. A great snack if you get hungry — loaded in vitamin C, fiber, and natural sugars — a pick-me-up with perks. The Romans ate them, so do I, and so should you.

Probiotics

Probiotics is a home-run-hitting category of nutritional supplements now found everywhere. Found in yogurt, these good bacteria support your flora, the good bacteria in your gastrointestinal tract, thereby preventing a myriad of problems. Now, there is a new category, called prebiotics — substances that fertilize the good bacteria in the gastrointestinal tract and encourage growth. Roughly 85% of the bacteria in our gastrointestinal tracts are the good guys and 15% the bad guys that cause human disease, and that ratio needs to be maintained.

The good bacteria make folic acid and vitamin K, along with lactic acid, H2O2 (hydrogen peroxide), and bacteriocins, nature's natural antibiotics. These chemicals keep the bad bacteria at bay.

Probiotics are indicated for irritable bowel syndrome, urinary tract infections with prolonged antibiotic use (over two weeks), decreased immunity with repeated infections, and vaginosis. Vaginosis in women presents with a malodorous vaginal discharge, caused by anaerobic bacteria, such as gardenella. With these peculiar bacteria, only certain antibiotics will work like clindamycin. The dose for the probiotic is brand determined, and as an addendum, it is now believed that our appendix may be a natural major producer of probiotics, which means you should leave it in if not a problem (acute appendicitis).

Pregnenolone

Pregnenolone has many, many actions because it makes many other things. Made in the adrenal gland, it lends a hand with production of sex hormones, DHEA, cortisol, aldosterone, epinephrine, and norepinephrine. It peaks around the age of twenty to thirty, and then starts tapering off.

1. Increases mood elevation and memory.
2. Decreases GABA receptor activity in the brain, which also helps with mood elevation.
3. Increases muscle mass in patients with wasting diseases called *sarcopenia.*
4. Increases blood pressure in patients who get dizzy because their blood pressures are too low. Shy-Drager syndrome presents with these symptoms with low blood pressures and pregnenolone works well.
5. Releases testosterone, helping men with low "T" syndrome, impotency, and erectile dysfunction.
1. The dose is 100-300 mg/day with indications of sexual dysfunction, low blood pressure, wasting diseases, and depression. Because it is steroid derived, long-term use can lead to fluid retention, diabetes, osteoporosis, and hypertension.

Horse chestnut

Horse chestnut needs to be primarily thought of as 'below the waist.'

1. Increases venous tone and vascular activity while also maintaining the connective tissue in the legs.
2. Decreases inflammation in the veins.

Indications include: varicose veins, venous stasis disease, and lymph edema. Lymph or brawny edema is swelling of the legs or arms that does not pit when pushed on by your finger. The other edema is called pitting edema where a finger imprint is left behind. They are different and have clinical implications, but with horse chestnut, the treatment is the same. The dose is brand-directed and it works despite the name.

Feverfew

Feverfew has a long history, dating back to the 17th Century for the treatment of migraine headaches. Its ingredients are the same as in turmeric or curcumin.

1. Increases the utilization of sugar in the brain.
2. Controls serotonin release and blood vessel activity in the brain.

In 1988, the British Journal *Lancet* reported feverfew decreased the severity and frequency of migraine headaches. Adding magnesium may help, but look for brands that include it. The indication is migraine headache and the dose is brand-directed. Remember, butterbur is also very effective in preventing and treating migraines and is much better. Since the medications we use for migraines are expensive and have many side effects, to use this and butterbur to treat migraines may make more sense.

Iron

Iron-deficient anemia has been with us for a long time. Fatigue and tiredness are its cardinal symptoms, with poor intake, digestive problems, and chronic bleeding as its causes. The most common cause in women is bleeding secondary to their menstrual periods. Hardly pathological, but when this occurs, iron needs to be replaced if low. Anemia is characterized as a small, red blood cell and low red color, which is generally the first clue. Red meat and green leafy vegetables have adequate amounts, so be sure to consume them. One warning: iron-deficient anemia in a non-menstruating female or male over the age of forty is cancer of the colon until proven otherwise and must be ruled out.

The indication for taking it is an iron-deficient blood level, low ferritin level, and an increased iron-binding capacity blood level. Treatment includes replacement with ferrous sulfate, 300 mg two to three times a day, which can cause gastric irritation; take it with food. Again, as a final warning: *do not* replace iron unless you are truly iron deficient (diagnosed via blood tests) and are negative for any gastrointestinal problems (bleeding). The bleeding in these instances is chronic, over a long period of time, and many times cannot be seen visibly in the stool. People with polyps, for example, will do this, and 85% of them will grow into cancer. Ah, that word "prevention" again!

Calcium
=======

True calcium deficiency is rare because our bones are a giant warehouse of it. If the serum levels drop, we automatically absorb it from bone to normalized blood levels. A low calcium level in our blood may not indicate a true calcium deficiency since a low albumin or protein level will artificially lower it. In the case of osteoporosis, women need 1500 g/day of calcium with vitamin D3 (5,000 i.u./day) at supper; not calcium carbonate since only 20% of it is absorbed. Any other calcium salt is acceptable, like calcium citrate. More recently, strontium and boron has been added to the regimen, strengthening the bones.

As a precaution, premenopausal women should be taking 1200 mg of calcium with vitamin D3 and postmenopausal women 1500 mg/day of calcium with D3 (5,000 i.u./day) either as supplements or milk/yogurt (250-300 g) per serving. Again, strontium and boron should be added. A true calcium deficiency needs calcium replacement to avoid muscle spasms, and a true elevated calcium level needs to be lowered to avoid coma, generally caused by parathyroid disease or bone metastasis from cancer.

Before you start treating calcium problems, you need to find out why yours is not normal. That's what your doctor is for. Ask him for an explanation in layman's terms so you can understand.

Wheat Grass

I'm an internist and a gastroenterologist, so it does my heart good to see nutrients make an appearance that are directed to the gastrointestinal tract. We don't know what causes inflammatory colitis like Ulcerative Colitis and Crohn's disease, but we do know that inflammation plays a very, very big role. These conditions are different pathologically, but inflammation is still the basic mechanism. Generally, they present with abdominal pain, diarrhea, and rectal bleeding and are considered systemic diseases because they will affect other organ systems like the skin, eyes, joints, and blood. Because we don't know what causes them, we are left with symptomatic treatment and, yes, the inflammation. Nutrients have been shown to help with the inflammation, like the omega-3 oils, mung bean extract, peony extract, curcumin, iron, vitamin B12, probiotics, Zyflamend and folic acid. Because the intestinal lining cells are metabolically active, their DNA must be supported, and don't forget about those mitochondria. We now know that in the gastrointestinal tract, inflammation of the lining cells can be tempered with butyrate found in wheat grass and phlorizin from apples. With the normalization of the inflammation, it may also prevent mutations of their cellular DNA that could prevent cancer.

Wheat Grass, a form of barley, is ancient and perhaps the first grass consumed by humans. Meaning, it has withstood the test of time and includes the following:

1. Full of vitamins, minerals, and beta carotene.
2. Contains anti-inflammatory saponarins and chlorophyll, which help neutralize TNF (a strong inflammatory) along with protecting fibroblasts against carcinogens —all inflammatory based. .
3. The younger and greener the grass the better. Just like green tea, with aging, even in plants, nutrients are diminished through oxidation as they age.
4. Studies in humans have shown wheat grass is an immune and inflammatory modulator. It increases chemical levels in the stool that normalize cell division to avoid cancer (as do apples and mung bean extract). Zinc may also help and has been shown to be effective in other inflammatory conditions, such as arthritis to help reduce arthritic symptoms. Again, it modulates down the inflammatory reaction, even in RA patients, who are the hardest to treat.
5. Since we know it can affect rapidly dividing cells, it should not surprise us that it can affect the bone marrow. It turns out wheat grass increases WBC (white blood cells) counts. In patients with low WBC counts, this can be very handy. It has already been shown to protect the bone marrow against the effects of

chemotherapy, like a depressed white cell count. Neupogen, a drug we frequently use, is an expensive medication that raises white blood cell counts and does the same thing. Wheat grass is also handy in treating other conditions like aplastic anemias, where the bone marrow just shuts down and does not make the WBCs.

6. Colitis patients, in a controlled study, had diminished symptoms of abdominal pain, diarrhea, and rectal bleeding of 78%, compared to 30% improvement in control patients with no wheat grass.

The normal dose is 15 mg a day taken with meals as either tablets or a juice. You can grow your own, but be careful about bacterial and fungal contamination since it needs a warm, moist environment. In my experience with colitis patients, if it is not severe, this along with the omega-3 oils, B12, folate, probiotic, iron, peony extract, and mung bean extract will be enough to control the symptoms and avoid the standard medications. Even if the standard medications are necessary, you will use less of them, saving money and reducing the risk of more severe side effects.

Caution: if you have true celiac disease with a positive biopsy of the small intestine, positive blood tests for it, or both, you cannot take the wheat grass. It's contraindicated. My approach to colitis is to start low with nutrients and then go higher with standard medications depending on the stubbornness of it, other systemic involvement (other body parts involved), and seriousness of the condition. That only makes sense. Remember, the stronger the medication, the more side effects and expense.

As an afterthought, and mentioned earlier, peony, with its immune modulator effect, may also be of help with Crohn's disease and ulcerative colitis, especially with severe cases.

Chapter Eleven

Cancer

Introduction

The second most common cause of death in this country is cancer. Our new understanding of its risk factors and how nutritional supplements help to prevent and treat it go a long way in dealing with cancer issues.

What is cancer, is a complicated question. Simply put, cancer is an abnormal assembly of cells that lack growth control, multiplied haphazardly, spread beyond their primary area (metastasis), and kills by organ failure or sepsis (infection). Genetics (family history), toxins (smoking, alcohol, and chemicals), chronic inflammation, and free radicals from any source are some of its known causes.

As a cancer survivor myself (kidney cancer), I can attest that a complete physical every year is your best defense — prevention is key.

Cancer can involve the solid organs or blood cells, as in leukemia and myeloma, and treatment may include: surgical removal, chemotherapy, radiation, and nutrients that can and should be used in tandem with standard medical therapy. We've already discussed some nutrients that can help prevent and treat cancer, but there are others. The emphasis here is finding ways to increase immunity ("T" cells) to kill the cancer cells, and genetic engineering.

Turmeric (curcumin)

A rhizome (root) from Asia and India (Ayurvedic), this volatile oil has been used for thousands of years. Found in many foods from India with a yellow color (like curry), its main actions are anti-inflammation and anti-cancer. MD Anderson Cancer Hospital's Cytokine Laboratory reported that 85% of colon cancer could potentially be prevented by using turmeric (curcumin) because it interrupted NFkB. By doing this, it prevented long-term inflammation in the colon cells from occurring. And since resveratrol does the same, I use them together for this reason.

1. Works to stop cancer cell development through cell-signaling pathways that normalize and regulate the growth of cells.
2. Maintains cell replication through all four stages and prompts tumor-suppression pathways that trigger death of tumor tissues.
3. Interferes with tumor invasion and blocks molecules that otherwise would open pathways to spread to other tissues.
4. Noninflammable affects in cervical cancer breaks the link, triggering the HPV (human papilloma virus) induced cancer.
5. Decreases bile salts that lead to colon cancer and inhibits gastric cancer cells from growing.
6. Reduces the rate of mutation.
7. Lowers cholesterol 21%, LDL (bad cholesterol) 43%, and increases HDL (good cholesterol) 50%.

8. Decreases blood sugar even more effectively than metformin, a drug we use for diabetes. It increases insulin receptor cells' membranes and, therefore, increases insulin binding capacity while blocking AGE products and oxidation effects of the diabetes. Sign me up!
9. Eases, in topical application, generalized skin inflammation.
10. Minor benefits for arthritis with its anti-Cox-2 activity, like arthritis medications. Decreases acid production for ulcer patients and decreases gas and bloating. My guess is it probably does this by decreasing stomach inflammation.

Indications include: cancer prevention, heart disease, stomach problems, diabetes, elevated lipids, arthritis, skin inflammation, and any inflammatory condition in the body at large, ulcer problems, and general medical care. The dose is brand-directed. The added plus is eating all the Indian food with curry in it that you can.

Selenium

Its story begins at the University of Arizona where in the early 90s, they embarked on a study looking at selenium's ability to prevent skin cancer. As it turned out, it had no effect on skin cancer, but it decreased lung-cancer rates so dramatically that the study was terminated early to publish the results.

1. Makes glutathione (a long acting antioxidant) and incorporates itself into other proteins for skin and nails.
2. Reacts like antioxidant enzymes that increase immunity, repair DNA, and help detoxify heavy metals like iron and mercury.

3. Helps with not only lung cancer, but cancer of the breast and prostate, too.
4. Has cardiovascular benefits by delaying fatty-acid oxidation and restoring the elasticity of our blood vessels.
5. Helps prostaglandins that will increase blood flow.
6. Helps with fertility and energy production as well.

Selenium reacts well with vitamin E and poorly with vitamin C, so make sure it *does* have vitamin E in it, but *no* vitamin C in any preparation you buy. Indications are those of cancer (prostate and breast) risks, general medical care, chronic fatigue, infertility, cardiovascular disease, heavy-metal exposure, with the dose 200-400 mcg/day in combination with vitamin E. You may still read of how selenium may cause bleeding; not true, ignore it.

Indole 3 Carbinol (13C)

As I mentioned earlier, Indole 3 Carbinol or 13C goes back to the beta-carotene story. This chemical found in cruciferous vegetables (cauliflower, cabbage, garden cress, bok choy, broccoli, Brussel sprouts, and similar green leafy vegetables) has been studied in relationship with beta carotene, sulforaphane, apigenin, and BITC (benzyl isothiocyanate).

1. These four horsemen of the cancer apocalypse induce phase one (help recognize the cancer cells to be eliminated), and detoxify estrogen and increase its excretion, so it won't drive potential cancer cells. More recent data suggests it may

help prevent and treat cervical cancer in women with the papilloma virus.

2. Maintains the ratio of the weak estrone (a steroid, a weak estrogen, and a minor female sex hormone) as compared to the stronger estradiol, like soy and green tea, which is beneficial in the prevention and treatment of breast cancer.
3. Beneficial effects on cervical and prostate cancer cells.
4. Scavenges free radicals, and many times you will find preparations containing rosemary to help with the antioxidative process.
5. Improves lupus, along with peony extract, DHEA, mung bean extract, and pregnenolone.

Indications include: prevention and treatment of colon cancer, cervical, breast, prostate cancers, lupus, and general medical care, with the dose brand-directed. Look for products with apigenin, BITC, and sulforaphane.

Apigenin

According to Harvard University, this may be only good guy found in cruciferous vegetables that decreases the cancer risk. Common sense tells us the things already mentioned, i.e., BITC, sulforaphane, and indole-3-carbinol, must be used in combination with it.

1. Prevents damage from inflammation with inhibition of NFkB.
2. Increases cancer cell death.
3. Inhibits new blood vessels for cancer growth with ovarian cancer cells and its cell proliferation.
4. Decreases vital carbohydrate transport to pancreatic cancer cells thereby starving them.

Indications: cancer prevention, i.e., ovarian, pancreas, and colon, with dose brand-directed. It would be a good idea also to eat all the cruciferous vegetables you can.

The natural way!

BITC (beta isothiocyanate)

Found in cruciferous vegetables, its chemical nature and indications are the same to the prior ones, all the cruciferous vegetables. Some of its actions are different but complimentary to the others.

1. Increases programmed cell death by signaling molecules that tell cancer it is time to close-up shop and die.
2. Shuts down and arrests the cycle to prevent replication of tumor cells.
3. Binds to the muscle-like intracellular proteins, thereby decreasing cell division in cancer cells.
4. Inhibits several cancer-promoting enzymes.
5. Produces butyrate levels in the colon, as do mung bean extract, apple skin extract, and wheat grass, preventing colon cancer and decreasing inflammation for treatment of colitis.

Indications: cancer prevention of the lung, breast, and colon, along with inflammatory colitis (ulcerative, Crohn's disease) in combination with 13C, apigenin, and sulforaphane, with the dose brand-directed.

Sulforaphane

Also found in cruciferous vegetables, it, too, prevents and fights cancer.

1. Targets specifically cancer stem cells. There was a substantial reduction in them without affecting normal cells.
2. Cancer cells treated with sulforaphane, when transplanted into other mice, failed to grow tumors.
3. Chinese studies in Oidong Province found a toxin called aflatoxin, derived from fungus, that causes liver cancer was prevented from causing DNA damage with Brussel sprouts with high levels of sulforaphane.

Indications again include: cancer prevention with dose brand-directed. Obviously, eat plenty of cruciferous veggies and look for supplements with all these things in them because they are now commercially available. In patients with a family history of colon cancer or patients with a history of polyps, they are a must, along with apple extract. Patients also with ulcerative colitis and Crohn's disease, because their accelerated inflammation, would do well to use them. With the inflammation of course, resveratrol, and curcumin are great add-ons.

Beta Sitosterol

Part of the plant steroid-like chemical complex, it is derived from soy and its main actions are directed to the prostate gland.

1. Increases cancer cell death.
2. Decreases prostaglandin synthesis, interrupting inflammation.
3. Neutralizes ROS, a very bad free radical.
4. Inhibits 5-alpha reductase that converts inactive testosterone to its active counterpart and enlarges the prostate.

5. Makes available to the prostate higher levels of pygeum africanum and stinging nettles, shrinking the prostate.
6. Increases urine flow and prevents the prostate from growing further over eighteen months.

It works with saw palmetto in good combination to increase urine flow while decreasing inflammation of the prostate, shrinking it. The indications are the prevention and treatment of prostate cancer along with BPH (benign prostate hypertrophy). The dose is brand-directed and used in combination with saw palmetto, soy protein, lycopene, EPA oils, green tea, selenium with vitamin E, and Zyflamend. Nice and tight, the combo works. If you ever have seen those commercials with Joe Theisman, the ex-football player, running from one port-o-potty to another, they are advertising sitosterol.

Maitake Mushrooms

There are over 20,000 different types of mushrooms, and about fifty have been found to have medicinal benefits. The best three are maitake, reishi, and shitake. At this point with maitake, our understanding is still very preliminary as compared to reishi mushrooms, but it is a start.

1. Benefits diabetes by lowering insulin resistance and improving blood sugars.
2. Benefits cardiovascular problems in general but only of secondary use.
3. Strong anti-cancer properties.
4. Prostate and breast tumors may benefit in not only helping to prevent these tumors but also help treat them.

5. For prostate cancer, many times I will add this on to the previous cocktail (above). For breast cancer, I use soy, green tea, EPA oils, selenium with vitamin E, and 13C, depending on how grave the problem is. Eating them as a food may help, but no studies have been ever done to prove it. The dose is brand-directed.

Quercetin

The expression, "An apple a day keeps the doctor away!" was well suited for quercetin. Quercetin is found not only in apples in large quantities, including the skin, but also in red wine, onions, grapefruit, green tea, vegetables, and beans. Its main effects are those of anti-inflammation and anti-allergy. A brief review of some of its important physiology, will help you understand in how it works. Since we know many cancers begin with inflammation, quercetin would be a logical way to prevent it.

Here's how:

1. Blocks the pro-inflammatory chemicals that lead to allergy and asthma.
2. Increases nitric oxide synthase (NOS), increasing nitric oxide and blood flow and improving circulation.
3. Decreases fat stores.
4. Prevents the release of histamines (antihistamine) and, therefore, decreases allergy.
5. Helps to decrease viral replication through its immune response.
6. Mimics calorie restriction, seen in yeast, to increase life span. Here, four genes are activated related to it.

A Korean study in 2007 found the production of inflammatory chemicals was decreased by blocking NFkB with quercetin; another example of why it works when treating allergies or asthma. The dose is 50-500 mg/day, but make sure to eat plenty of apples with the skin on. Other good things in apples include chlorogenic acid, like we find in coffee, to prevent and treat diabetes and phloridzin, which increases colon butyrate levels to prevent colon cancer.

Indications include: allergy, asthma, migraine headaches, arthritis, decreased immunity, general medical care, risk factors for cancer, e.g., family history, and coronary artery disease.

Just as in red wine, many other uses will be found in the future for quercetin. When eating an apple, eat the skin and the fruit, but not the seeds. They have cyanide in them.

Vitamin D3 (not Vitamin D2)

For years, Dr. E. Giovannucci at Harvard has been saying vitamin D3 will decrease cancer risks. Everyone criticized him, but guess what? He was correct. We now know if your Vitamin D3 level is low, your risk of cancer of the colon, esophagus, pancreas, and ovary increases approximately 50%.

We also thought the twenty minutes of sun provided enough vitamin D3 through the skin's metabolism, thinking we did not have to supplement it, but we were wrong. Not only that, we, in the medical profession, told people not to drink milk because the fat in it presented a risk of heart disease — wrong, again. In doing all these things, we created a whole society who is now deficient in vitamin D3, along with calcium and conjugated linoleic acid (CLA) that prevents cancer and helps with weight loss.

As I mentioned, it had also been erroneously stated that only twenty minutes in the sun was sufficient for vitamin D3 absorption — another inaccurate presumption. I screen all my patients for vitamin D3 levels, and even people who work outside all day in the Florida sun have low levels. Now, if they have low levels, I would hate to see the levels of patients from the northern states where the sun exposure is much less. How about Seattle, huh?

There have been many misconceptions and incorrect assumptions concerning vitamin D3. We know vegetarians will become deficient in vitamin B12, but also vitamin D3. Another error from the medical profession has been understating the recommended dosage. For years, and even today, 400 i.u./day is recommended, but the corrected dose is 5,000 i.u./day and it must be D3, not D2, or 25 OH Cholecalciferol; read the label. Lastly, since it is fat soluble, better blood levels can be achieved if taken at meals with other fats.

1. Allows for absorption of calcium from bone and the gastrointestinal tract to maintain calcium blood levels, but has no effect on reabsorbing calcium from the kidney. This closed circuit keeps our calcium levels within a very tight range and is very efficient. You can see as an aside that any disease affecting the GI tract, kidneys, and bone could have a profound effect on calcium levels in either direction. If calcium is too high, you will go into a coma, and if too

low, you will develop muscle spasms and tetani due to deficiency.

2. Regulates cell genes through division, differentiation, proliferation, programmed cell death, and the formation of new blood vessels; a clear link to cancer concerning prevention.

3. May help decrease sugar levels because there are vitamin D3 receptors in cells of the pancreas where insulin is produced. The supposition would be then, it helps produce and release insulin.

4. Decreased vitamin D3 levels were associated with a two and one-half times increased risk of heart attack.

5. Helps drop influenza rates and other viral problems.

6. The *Archives of Internal Medicine* reported patients with normal levels of vitamin D3 had a 7% less mortality overall than those with low levels; a simple enough statement with profound implications.

7. Low levels of vitamin D3 have recently been linked to Parkinsonism.

The dose is 5000 i.u./day and the indications include: cancer prevention, increase immunity, general medical care, osteoporosis, Parkinsonism, and coronary artery disease or its risk factors. Diabetes could also be a consideration since there are vitamin D receptors in the pancreas, but more data is needed.

Don't depend on the sun or the medical profession at large. Drink milk and get your vitamin D blood level checked every year.

Resveratrol

Resveratrol is found not only in red grapes and red wine, but also grape juice, peanuts, berries, and pine nuts.

1. The chemistry of the red grape is astonishing, with phytoalexins, saponins, sirtuin, and polyphenols, such as proanthocyanidins and flavonoids.
2. Studies have shown resveratrol increased life spans by 70%.
3. A University of Virginia study found its ability to decrease NFkB (inflammation) is consistent with a study in the *European Journal of Pharmacology* that reported colitis-induced animals had a 40% higher mortality when not given resveratrol as compared to the study group on resveratrol.
4. In the *Journal of Endocrinology and Metabolism*, its anti-inflammatory actions included a reduction in ROS (the big, bad free radical), TNF, interleukin-6, and C reactive protein, which we commonly used to measure inflammation in our bodies. If they are high, then there is active inflammation.
5. Resveratrol also turns on the stem cells of the endothelial lining cells of our blood cells. Now how incredible can it be, that it repairs blood vessels by stimulating adult stem cells? It's your own, personal stem-cell transplant.
6. Decreases cholesterol, plaque, and abnormal heart rhythms, and lowers blood pressure by decreasing angiotensin 2, which is responsible for fibrosis of the heart, leading to diastolic dysfunction and congestive heart failure. This diastolic dysfunction means that the heart can't fill properly and, in doing so, the ejection fraction will be lower leading to shortness of

breath and heart failure. Carnitine, lipoic acid, branched chain amino acids and taurine I recommend, along with the resveratrol, for this reason.

7. Increases insulin sensitivity by affecting the cells mitochondria, which may also be affected by sirtuins to lower blood sugars.

8. May lower the proliferation of breast, prostate, stomach, colon, pancreas, and thyroid cancers.

Clinical studies have shown it to enhance cancer-cell sensitivity to an immune death. A study by the University of Alabama found an eight-fold decrease in prostate cancer by using supplements of resveratrol comparable to drinking eight liters per day of red wine. Take the supplement. Another study showed red-wine consumption decreased colon-cancer rates by 68% and white wine by 0%, while the *Journal of Carcinogenesis* found it decreased breast cancer.

The dose is generally 20 mg/day and is brand determined along with drinking red wine. My recommendation is two glasses of red wine for men and one for women with dinner. More than one drink of alcohol per day in women increases the risk of breast cancer. I recommend resveratrol be combined with pterostilbene to help turn on and turn off certain genes we will discuss shortly. The dose is brand-directed and indications include: cancer, diabetes, HBP, chronic inflammation, congestive heart failure, all other cardiac diseases, lipid elevation, and general medical care.

Pterostilbene

Found in blueberries and grapes (sound familiar?), it generally is harvested from the Indian Kino tree.

Pterostilbene is structurally and biochemically like resveratrol, so it is easy to see how pterostilbene and resveratrol work together synergistically.

1. Together, they activate the longevity gene, in the same manner that calorie restriction does. For example, resveratrol activates the beginning of molecular cascades by turning on the good genes, while Pterostilbene affects the latter molecules by turning off the bad ones.
2. They do the same thing with cancer, turning on programmed cell death, and turning off genes to prevent metastasis and invasion of other tissues.
3. Pterostilbene, by itself, suppresses genes involved with inflammation, and in cancers it inhibits genes that make molecules allowing cancer cells to stick to vessel walls, therefore making them vulnerable to immune attack and death.
4. Suppresses pre-cancerous cells in the colons of carcinogenic-exposed animals, and prevented cancer cells from communicating with each other through special connections called 'gap junctions.'
5. Prevents the loss of dopamine neurotransmitters having to do with memory centers (NMDA receptors). Clinically, in aged animals, who'd been given blueberries and pterostilbene, memory improved in three weeks; a direct link to the activation of brain signal proteins of the hippocampus.

The dose is brand-determined, with resveratrol added. Get the supplement; 30 mg of pterostilbene equals 140 cups of blueberries! Indications include: the same as resveratrol, i.e., general medical care., cancer, CNS and brain dysfunction, cardiovascular and lipid problems, chronic inflammation, and probably diabetes. Look for resveratrol with pterostilbene in it; another "two-fer."

Saw Palmetto

Native to New Zealand, France, Germany, and Austria, this plant is becoming scarce because of its medicinal popularity. When you think of saw palmetto, you think of the prostate gland, which effects both enlargement and cancer. Testosterone is normally made in the testicles and secreted into the blood stream, and must be acted on by 5 alpha reductases to become active (25 hydroxydihydrotestosterone). Unfortunately, it is also acted on by aromatase in the blood stream and converted to estrogen, creating a problem with the low testosterone syndrome we see in men with loss of libido, erectile dysfunction, large breasts, and other related symptoms.

1. Interferes with *both* enzyme converters, with studies showing a decrease in urine symptoms, increased flow, and an increase in function.
2. In prostatic hypertrophy, urine outflow is obstructed and symptoms of frequent urination, especially at night, occur. The bladder never empties completely and, as a result, you must go every thirty minutes.
3. Acts on the alpha 1 receptor like the drugs Cardura and Flomax, to increase urine flow without raising the PSA (prostatic specific antigen, a marker for cancer) level.
4. More effective when used with pygeum africanum, pumpkin seed, and stinging nettles; look for brands with them in it.

The dose is brand-directed and indications include: BPH (benign prostatic hypertrophy) and cancer of the prostate (prevention and treatment). One more thing, since saw palmetto blocks 5 alpha reductase, it may help with balding since Propecia, a drug used for this, does the same thing. A little medical secret, Propecia is the same thing as Proscar, a drug we use for prostate problems but at a lower dose.

Lycopene

A red pigment found in things like tomatoes, red peppers, grapefruit, and watermelon, it is part of the carotenoid family. This chemical is fat soluble, meaning, when consumed, it is absorbed if a fat present, such as tomatoes on pizza with cheese. The converse is also true. If you drink a glass of tomato juice by itself, the lycopene will not be absorbed, so have some cheese and crackers with it. In addition, when food with lycopene in it is heated, i.e. tomatoes, more is released and available to you. So, cook it.

1. Because of the red color and a high antioxidant level, we know it must be good for us.
2. Helps the detoxification of drugs and chemicals in the blood.
3. Helps to prevent oxidation of lipids.
4. Decreases the risk of prostate cancer.
5. Increases immunity, therefore decreasing infection rates and cancer.
6. Helps with the treatment of macular degeneration.
7. Decreases cancer along with asthma and sunburn damage.
8. May decrease osteoporosis and arteriosclerotic heart disease.

The dose is 15 mg/day, and indications include: osteoporosis, macular degeneration, cardiovascular disease and their risk factors, prostate cancer for prevention and treatment, and BPH. More recently, lycopene has been shown to protect the skin (against the sun) whether it be in pill form or a lycopene cream. The cream is especially good for any inflammatory skin problems.

This I use many times in conjunction with soy protein, saw palmetto, beta sitosterol, vitamin E/selenium, green tea, EPA, and Zyflamend for prostate-related problems.

Growth Hormone

Also known as GH, somatotropin, IGF (insulin growth factor), and somatomedin-C, it is made in the pituitary part of the brain, and mainly responsible for growth. Once we have reached our maximum growth, its role in human physiology becomes a bit murky.

1. Dr. Rudman at the University of Wisconsin studied growth hormone in adults over six months and found it affected lean body mass and fat tissue, influencing ten to twenty years of aging.
2. Taken up by the liver, it binds to cells including the brain while increasing insulin sensitivity and decreasing fat.
3. Builds more bone, muscle, and nerves, both central and peripheral, and there seems to be "bursts" of activity during sleep with levels going up, then returning to normal quickly.
4. May be related to chronic diseases, like amyotrophic lateral sclerosis (ALS) or Lou

Gehrig's disease, by improving or delaying the disease process.

5. Prevents arteriosclerosis, reverses arterial plaque by increasing the HDL (good cholesterol), and decreasing the LDL (bad cholesterol) and diastolic blood pressure.

6. May have a "Lazarus Effect" described by Frank Herbert, the writer of *Dune,* where you go from low self-esteem, anxiety, and depression to a 'wake up' state.

7. Increases immunity by increasing "T" cell function through the thymus gland, therefore, preventing virus and cancer.

8. Improves lung function with an increase in oxygen and exercise tolerance.

9. Increases bone density to improve osteoporosis.

10. Sexual studies have not been done, but you could probably guess its effects with sexual dysfunction (decreased libido and erectile dysfunction).

11. Improves brain function with an increase in focus and concentration.

12. Re-contours the body by decreasing fat and increasing muscle.

The dose of growth hormone will depend on blood levels and can only be given under the tongue or by injection. My choice is the former, under the tongue; cheaper and safer.

Indications include: general medical care, heart disease, immune impairment, muscle weakness, osteoporosis, COPD (chronic obstructive lung disease, i.e. emphysema), weight loss, chronic fatigue, early dementia, and perhaps Lou Gehrig's disease. Depression and sexual dysfunction may benefit, but more studies need to be done. Please, do not be duped into claims from the growth hormone clinics that promise you the world and optimal health for a small fortune (yours). Talk to your physician first. A great body requires more than just growth hormone.

Chapter Twelve

Lung Disease, Pycnogenol, and Coffee

Introduction

The lungs are a mine field for free radicals because that's where most of the oxidation occurs, and from a nutritional standpoint, we are just beginning to understand it. Hardening of the arteries is likewise related to oxidation at the blood-vessel level and will be reviewed.

Cysteine

An essential amino acid, we have used it for years for the mucous problems principally seen in cystic fibrosis patients (children and young adults). Lung diseases such as asthma and COPD (chronic obstructive lung disease, i.e., emphysema) really represent states of chronic inflammation and their long-term effects are just being realized.

Cysteine helps with many things:

1. Breaks apart mucous and helps to make an antioxidant that can neutralize ROS in the lungs.
2. May help with the overall aging process of the lungs with fibrosis, in that it affects oxidative stress and DNA throughout our body.

3. Generally used in conjunction with glutathione, a long-acting antioxidant made in the liver.

The dose is brand-directed and generally used for lung conditions, such as asthma, COPD, and emphysema, along with general medical care. Cysteine and glutathione, along with the drug Daliresp, are great ways to decrease inflammation in the lungs, thereby decreasing long-term damage. Again, to prevent is better than to treat. The other anti-inflammatories, like curcumin and resveratrol, can also be used in conjunction.

There is gathering evidence that excessive exercise puts an overload of free radicals in the lung that could lead to scarring and lung (pulmonary) fibrosis over the long term. A good example would be marathon runners, so keep that in mind if you like to jog. Lastly, the Mayo Clinic reported that in patients with ongoing inflammation not responding to the normal medications, if treated with Motrin, an anti-inflammatory drug, the lung condition improves. I rarely prescribe it for patients with respiratory infections that are not improving with the standard therapies.

Pycnogenol

This was discussed earlier, but because of its amazing antioxidant activity, I've resurrected it in the context of providing an "antioxidant bank" to help with scenarios, such as over exercising. Rising from the ashes like a giant Phoenix, pycnogenol just gets better and better. An extract from maritime bark, you can find it in grape seeds, peanut skins, and witch hazel.

1. Loaded with bioflavins and proanthocyanidins, it's stronger than green tea in regard to antioxidant activity.
2. Twenty-times more potent with antioxidants and as an anti-inflammatory than vitamin C and fifty times more potent than vitamin E. Even with ROS, the very strong free radicle, it decreases its inflammatory markers.
3. Prevents and reverses cardiovascular disease. In patients with coronary artery disease on pycnogenol, levels of oxidative stress showed just after eight weeks remarkable improvement in the lining of the blood vessels, whereas placebo levels were zero. With arterial disease, any improvement, not just maintaining status quo, is fantastic and will hopefully prevent many future problems and related costs. More recently, pycnogenol has been shown to benefit the neuropathy of diabetes with numbness in the legs, and does so by improving circulation through the tiny arteries (microvasculature).
4. Decreases in patients with congestive heart failure symptoms, such as shortness of breath, by 28% compared to just 14% in the placebo group.
5. Decreases blood pressure better than Altace, a good standard HBP medication, increases walking on the treadmill three times more than prior to therapy, and equates to better blood flow into the heart.

Now the $64,000 question: How does it do these things? Pycnogenol mechanisms are very basic, but it does them very well; a direct relation to its potency and usefulness especially with the 'antioxidant bank.'

Here are some of the basics:

1. Increases substances that in turn increase nitric acid and dilate blood vessels.
2. Decreases inflammation.
3. Decreases blockage of the flow of blood to the heart caused by a blood clot in a coronary artery.
4. Lowers blood sugar, but its main benefit is with the tiny blood vessels.
5. Improves ringing in the ears by increasing blood flow through the cochlear.
6. Hydrates and improves the elastic tissue of skin. Therefore, less wrinkles. Dark discolorations of the skin, especially of the face, improve with rub-on pycnogenol (like lycopene cream), which bleaches and prevents dark spots from getting darker.
7. Helps with venous stasis disease, restless leg syndrome, and dependent edema. These seem minor in comparison to the other effects, but if you have them, they can be disturbing.

In summary, we already know diabetes is not a sugar disease but an accelerated blood-vessel disease. It must be managed early to avoid the vascular consequences, such as peripheral vascular disease, a precursor to vascular insufficiency in the legs, neuropathies, gangrene, and diabetic leg ulcers. With heart and early coronary disease, it needs no explanation. Brain vascular events, like strokes in diabetics, have been well-established, and when we do brain scans on them, they show atrophic brains with the white matter being diminished. Therefore, its effect on decreasing microvascular inflammatory changes throughout the body is critical.

The first step is the inflammation of LDL at the blood-vessel wall level. Next come macrophages, because the inflammation engulfs the fatty cells, making them "foam cells." Smooth muscle cells in the blood-vessel lining then proliferate and "cap around" the plaque, stiffening the blood vessel and decreasing the blood flow. Pycnogenol is extremely effective because it interrupts *all* these steps at multiple levels.

As far as I am concerned, everyone should be on pycnogenol along with the omega-3/7 oils, AMPK (works like metformin), bilberry, green coffee extract, and carnosine to neutralize AGE particles. Again, nutrients can and should play a large role in treating all diabetics and aging.

The dose of pycnogenol can vary depending on the condition and the gravity of it but generally it is 100-200 mgs/day. It is relatively expensive, so don't be surprised, but it is not near the price of what most medications will cost you. Make sure you get a good brand as the results will depend on it, and its profound positive effects with diabetes and heart disease puts it in the category of anti-aging.

Coffee

Coffee has gotten a bad rap the past few decades, where it has been stated that coffee is bad for you and it can lead to gastric irritation and ulceration. The coffee part is wrong, but the irritation and ulceration is true. In addition, in the early '90s, Harvard published a study stating coffee may cause pancreatic cancer. Most definitely *not* true. Therefore, we must overcome these historical misnomers and move on.

Coffee is a fruit containing more than 1000 compounds. The major ones include polyphenols and chlorogenic acid. The chlorogenic acid, to a large extent, is destroyed with roasting, but enough is still left to do beneficial things. For years, there has been an ill-defined notion that coffee benefits diabetics, and it does. The average American consumes about one to three cups of coffee a day, so we will let that be our yardstick for benefit comparisons. Generally speaking, if you drink more than six cups of coffee per day you will live 10-15% longer. Research over the last few years tells us the following:

1. Coffee improves diabetes by 13% with one cup of coffee a day, 47% with four cups, and 67% with twelve cups per day. It is believed the chlorogenic acid interferes with glucose synthesis and glucose 6 phosphates that lower blood sugars, as does metformin, a drug we use to treat diabetics and AMPK, a nutrient.

2. Consuming coffee in certain amounts is directly related to decreasing certain cancer risks. For example, six cups of coffee relate to an 18% decrease of prostate cancer and 40% lower risk of the aggressive lethal prostate cancer. Five cups of coffee relate to a 57% decrease of the estrogen receptor negative type breast cancer; the harder one to treat. In colon cancer, heavy coffee consumers have a 30% decrease. The chlorogenic acid and the polyphenols protect the cell's DNA thereby preventing cellular transformation into cancers.

3. Perhaps the most exciting arena for coffee use is with dementia and Alzheimer's disease. Recent research has been reported that the polyphenols in coffee improve signaling proteins of the brain. Moreover, coffee, in sufficient amounts, protects primary neuronal cells and lowers beta and

gamma secretase used as markers for amyloid deposits in the brain we see in Alzheimer's disease. One study demonstrated five cups of coffee a day reversed early Alzheimer's disease in five weeks.

4. Since roasting destroys some of the chlorogenic acid, there is now a commercial brand extracted prior to roasting called green coffee extract. This delivers a much higher dose of the good guys, with the dose being 200 mgs two to three times a day. If you want to get the most out of regular coffee, soak the beans for twelve hours prior to making the coffee.

Indications include: diabetes mellitus, cancer prevention, general medical care, and treatment of dementias, including Alzheimer's disease.

Chapter Thirteen

Immunity and Cancer

I touched on immunity in chapter four with immunosenescense, but this is a multi-faceted issue. Let's go a bit deeper here into the immune system as it relates to the prevention and treatment of cancer.

The problem with nutrients is they do multiple things, which makes them difficult to classify. Drugs on the other hand are easier because they generally have one purpose only.

Many nutrients touch immunity, but of the more recent ones, zinc, enzymatically modified rice bran, reishi mushrooms, and cistanche are the most fascinating, so I'm going to group them together. We don't know yet if using them together adds benefit, but I would think so.

Zinc

We touched on it with the discussion of the common cold. A trace element, zinc was not thought to be very important until recently, unless you had anorexia or a wasting problem, where zinc deficiency is very common. But with new insights into immunosenescense, the specter of zinc has raised its head again. It turns out zinc is involved with 2000 nuclear cell activities and, subsequently, effects many biological functions.

1. Increases "T" cell (killer cell) function; necessary for the prevention and treatment of viral and fungal infections, and cancer.
2. Paradoxically, if zinc levels are low, the immune system is increased and sensitized as in the autoimmune diseases, i.e., lupus, scleroderma. So, when you think of zinc, think immunity, either not enough or too much.
3. Has a positive effect on cancer prevention and treatment. In animals with experimentally induced cancers, the ones with normal zinc levels had a 28% less incidence of cancer. Zinc has additionally been shown to increase cancer surveillance and starve cancer cells of carbohydrates, therefore not allowing them to grow. Non-Hodgkin's lymphoma patients with normal zinc levels have a 42% lower incidence.
4. Reduces the level of a tumor growth promoter in prostate cancer patients. Normally, the prostate contains high levels of zinc as compared to other tissues (ten times), but with cancer, the levels decrease. Zinc, therefore, decreases the cancer risk from spreading. Research on blood levels of zinc and its effect on cancer is just beginning and there will be much more coming because, again, it makes sense regarding its profound effects on DNA.

Zinc should only be used in doses of 50 mg/day or less. If you use larger doses, you will become copper deficient, then that, too, must be replaced. Anemia, low white cell counts, bone fractures, diabetes, and arrhythmias can result. If you do use doses greater than 50 mg/day, then add copper, 2 mg/day.

Food can help. A normal serving of oysters provides 74 mg, beef chuck roasts 7 mg. You can get zinc from plant sources, but cereals, breads, and legumes can bind it and prevent its absorption.

In summary, get your zinc levels checked. It is not a standard test/part of a normal blood screen, so you will have to ask for it.

Enzymatically Modified Rice Bran

If you remember the basics when it comes to immunity, the "T" cells are separated into two groups. The "innate" ones are the immediate responders, while the "adaptive" ones are delayed, many times requiring antibody attachment first because they need to be programmed on what to do. Reishi mushrooms stimulate the innate-immediate ones, while cistanche stimulate the adaptive-delayed ones, making them the perfect combination.

Enzymatically modified rice bran has been found to stimulate the innate-immediate ones. This is what we know thus far:

1. Increases innate cells by 84% in old mice five-fold in just two days.
2. Helps stimulate the immune system in older people.
3. Fights against the herpes viruses seen in chronic fatigue syndrome, i.e. Epstein-Barr and Cytomegalic.
4. Increases cell death in tumor cells.
5. Increases "B" cell numbers, too, and helps control the inflammatory cytokines. The problem with this is because of the overstimulation it causes, it can only be used for three-to-four

months. Great in combination with reishi mushrooms and cistanche. I use them commonly for the treatment of chronic fatigue syndrome, fibromyalgia, low immune states, and cancer prevention and treatment.

Cistanche

A Chinese remedy going back at least 1000 years, Cistanche is a yellow-flowered plant, and its main role is the immune system. Its active ingredient stimulates the adaptive ones that many times require an antibody to hook onto the "bad guys" to destroy them. That's called opsonization. Here you can see the intimate relationship of the "B" and "T" cells, who need each other, but as we get older this system fades and we become more susceptible to viruses, bacteria, and cancer.

1. Increases helper cells and decreases suppressor cells seen in AIDS patients, and increases our immunity to the virus.
2. Wakens memory cells to ward off viruses, like the one that causes chronic fatigue syndrome and fibromyalgia.
3. Increases growth hormone levels.

Cistanche is almost always used with reishi mushrooms and can be used for long periods of time, months, in fact. Their effects are very subtle, but in time, the viruses will stop replicating and all the symptoms will improve. Their short- and long-term effects on cancer prevention and treatment are being looked at currently, but I would advise that if you have any risk factors, take them. There is nothing to lose!

Reishi Mushrooms

Of the 20,000 different types of mushrooms, only a few have medicinal value and reishi is one of them.

1. Increases both "B" and "T" cell function.
2. Increases macrophages and dendritic cells, the first to encounter the "bad guys" and break them down to be processed by the "T" and "B" cells.
3. Affects the bone marrow itself in perpetuating these cell lines. They may, in fact, be utilizing stem cells; not only improving function of these cells but also increasing cell numbers.
4. Increases the adaptive cell line of "T" cells. These are the ones specialty programed for their anti-cancer, antibacterial, antifungal, antiviral activities. Cistanche and rice bran affects innate "T" cells, which work immediately.

Reishi does it all by increasing the actual numbers and effectiveness of "B" and "T" cells, while decreasing inflammation. I use it for chronic fatigue syndrome, immunosenescense, cancer prevention, or any serious infection.

Within the last six months, we have realized that worn out cells, near their termination, are released into the blood stream. They are called senescent cells and act like very active free radicles. The body normally clears them, but in some people, they are not cleared effectively and cause long term problems elsewhere in the body. Killer "T" cells are the primary clearing agents, but when not able, we need help. Recent studies have reported that vitamin B3 and resveratrol will remove these free radicle senescent cells and may help with unexplained inflammation or multi-system diseases. This, again, is another variant of aging and immune system failure.

Finally

Now regarding immunity, we have a game plan to prevent and treat all types of infections. This of course includes patients who are at risk for cancer and those who have it. Immune-compromised patients should be on these without question. The problem has been the reluctance of mainstream doctors agreeing to it because they have no knowledge of it.

Look at it this way, if you had cancer and there was a drug that would cure it, but your doctor was not aware of it, therefore denying you of a cure, would that be acceptable? In my opinion, there is no difference. Your doctor has a responsibility to stay current, not only with mainstream medicine but alternative therapies as well, and in this way can offer you many options and remedies. The oncologist and cardiologist whom I use welcome alternative therapies and have included them into their practice, but most other doctors have not been so understanding.

Chapter Fourteen

Honey and Foods of Great Nutritional Value

Introduction

It's amazing something ancient to us can also be relatively new. Honey, around since Egyptian times with Imhotep, has made a comeback, and now there is a variant. This is a good example of a dietary benefit from the foods we eat called nutraceuticals. Let's look at *it*, and more.

Honey

We earlier reviewed honey's ancient history along with its medicinal benefit as an antibacterial agent, especially with skin infections, but there is a new kid on the block from Africa and New Zealand called manuka. Manuka honey works much like regular honey regarding bacteria, viruses, inflammation, along with increasing immunity. It can be rubbed on or ingested, but it is also useful with sore throats, bites, bloody noses, skin lesions, and canker sores. These are small problems that can be very annoying, will not go away, and many times recur.

I have found Manuka very useful in bloody noses since most originate at the tip of the nose. Putting a fingertip full inside the anterior part of the nose will coagulate and stop the bleeding, then pinch the tip of the nose until the bleeding stops. Again, these problems are not life threatening, but can be very problematic.

When regular honey and manuka are compared to the topical antibiotics like Bactroban for skin infections, the honeys have better results.

Walnuts

What is the best nut nutritionally? The answer is walnuts, which are edible seeds, not nuts. There are three types, the English (Persian), which is the most common, black, and white. Walnuts are not only better than the rest but about twice as nutritious because of what is in them.

1. This powerful nut/seed contains vitamins, phenolic acids, flavonoids, phytosterols, and polyunsaturated oils.
2. Decrease hyperactivity of the brain, related to seizure activity and children's behavior, according to a study by Purdue University.
3. Oils in the walnuts decrease lipids and increase the elasticity of blood vessels, and, therefore, increase blood flow, stated the *American Journal of Clinical Investigation*.
4. Daily consumption of walnuts, along with vitamin E, may help prevent breast, prostate, and lung cancers. At the University of California at Davis, walnut extract decreased prostate cancer cell growth by 40% in mice. Along with this was Marshall University's data of the phytosterols (plant estrogen-like chemicals) in walnuts that filled estrogen receptor sites and, subsequently, decreased breast-cancer rates.

5. Improves the lining of blood vessel function responsible for blood flow in diabetics.
6. Decreases telopeptide levels, the measure of bone breakdown, protecting against osteoporosis, Penn State found. This was due to the walnuts' alpha linoleic acid, and occurred after just six weeks.
7. Decreases lipid levels and helps with weight loss Loma Linda University found.

Eat a handful of nuts every day and, if you don't mind walnuts, eat them because they are the best.

Cruciferous Vegetables

In the 1980s, studies began to suggest a diet high in fiber and cruciferous vegetables could prevent colon cancer. Beta carotene was the first to be studied, but the results were conflicting. If not beta carotene, what was in broccoli, kale, spinach, and the like that could tip the difference in preventing colon cancer? We now have a pretty good idea, and eating these vegetables or a nutrient supplement should solve the problem. But let's take another look at the chemicals in them. A review of chapter eleven will refresh your memory.

As discussed before, the first is apigenin, which Harvard University thinks may be the only one responsible and may be particularly involved in pancreatic and ovarian cancers.

1. In the pancreas, apigenin turns off vital sugar transfer into tumor cells, basically starving them to death.
2. It increases programmed cell death, preventing NFkB damage, and all decrease proliferation of the tumor cells.

3. In ovarian cancer, apigenin decreases new blood vessel growth, further inhibiting cell growth.

The second chemical we find in the cruciferous group is benzyl isothiocyanate (BITC); relevant with colon, breast, and lung cancers.

1. Increases programmed cell death.
2. Decreases cell division and inhibits several cancer-promoting cytochrome enzymes.

You notice these cruciferous chemicals can affect different tumors depending on the active ingredients, making their influence wider than you would expect.

Sulforaphane

1. Researchers at the University of Michigan reported in the *Journal of Clinical Cancer Research* that mice with breast cancer, when treated with sulforaphane, had a decrease in tumor size because it targeted the cancer stem cells.
2. In Oidong Province, China, where liver cancer is very common because of a fungus in peanuts called aflatoxin, it was found that the tea they drink from Brussel sprouts (cruciferous) containing apigenin decreased the urine markers for damaged DNA because of the fungus. Therefore, the apigenin from the Brussel sprouts stopped damage to the DNA.

Here again the advice would be for us to eat as much roughage and cruciferous vegetables as we can. Supplements are now available with all these active ingredients in them, but, of course, then you lose the important fiber. This may be the answer for those broccoli haters out there, but for most people, the truth would be in the middle. It is hard to not take note of the data, especially when the epidemiological studies thirty years ago confirm this. One thing's for sure, if a family history of colon cancer exists, or you have polyps, eat the veggies, take the supplement, and get those surveillance colonoscopies.

Peppermint

Did you ever go into a restaurant and as you were leaving, they gave you a mint? Now, why would they do that? To say, 'Thank you'? To improve your breath? The reason was to improve your digestion and make you more satisfied with the meal, enticing you to return. Pretty clever, don't you think? And a good reason exists for this thinking, even though it was an observation noted by chefs many years ago. Peppermint is a root containing menthol, limonene, caryophyllene, eucalyptus, pinene, and pulegone.

1. Contains high concentrations of the natural pesticide pulegone and for years has been used as a natural remedy for nausea, vomiting, sinus, colds, and increasing mental alertness.
2. Studies have ranged back to 2007, showing symptoms would improve 20-40% for mostly irritable bowel disease. In 2011, a study of irritable bowel disease patients showed the same but also noted a dramatic drop of abdominal pain symptoms they thought was due to a decrease in sensory channel TRPM 8. This is important and you will see it again.
3. Increased transit time was noted and made sense because we know irritable-bowel patients have

delayed transits. Normally, when you eat something, it takes two-four days to get to your rectum, while with irritable bowel disease, patients can have transit times of eight-ten days.
4. Decreases gas, spasms, and is antibacterial; quite beneficial when it comes to bacterial and viral gastroenteritis.

Peppermint can help with a myriad of conditions having to do with your gastrointestinal tract, from irritable bowel syndrome to infectious gastroenteritis. Benign enough to take with no side effects and has minimal costs.

Basil

There are over sixty varieties of basil coming from Africa and Asia. In Greek, the word basil means "royal" and for good reason. Ingredients include: vitamin K, calcium, oils, and beta caryophyllene, whose major effect is that of anti-inflammation.

1. The anti-inflammatory effects are due mostly to its Cox-2 activity, which we see in arthritis medications, and steroids. Knowing this, you would guess it would benefit arthritis and inflammatory colitis, like ulcerative and Crohn's disease, and it does.
2. Protects cellular DNA with two flavonoids.
3. Antibacterial because of the oils, including: astragal, cloves, rosmarinic, and linolool. An Iranian study reported basil inhibited staphylococcus, bacillus cereus, and E. coli. Bacillus cereus is the organism found in brown rice seen in sushi poisoning. Contrary to belief, it

is not always the raw fish but the rice that may make you sick.

4. Decreases both systolic and diastolic hypertension and relieves stress.

These are great reasons to use basil in your cooking, and, gratefully, is used a lot in the Mediterranean diet. I predict there will be more benefits found for it with caryophyllene in it. I'm beginning to see this chemical raise its head in other nutrients, so there must be real benefits we just haven't seen yet. Obviously, the anti-inflammatory and antibacterial effects are important, along with lowering blood pressure, too, since they work together in a synergistic way. Grow your own, as we do, and spice up your life and health. If you have any inflammatory condition, especially if chronic, I would consume it daily.

Red Peppers

Now this should be a no-brainer because of the color we are directed to. Yes, red, and how much more deliberate and obvious can it be. Besides vitamins A, E, B6, and C (twice as much as an orange), it has fiber and over thirty carotenoids. Lycopene, found in tomatoes and watermelon, alpha and beta carotene, cryptoxanthin, lutein, zeaxanthin, quercetin, caffeic acid, and apigenin are just a few, and some we have already discussed.

1. Helps prevent prostate, breast, and lung cancer. Obviously, the lycopene and apigenin are the main players here.
2. For our eyes due to the immense benefits derived from the carotenes, zeaxanthin, and lutein.

3. Caffeic acid in red peppers decreased blood sugars and reduced insulin resistance, according to a Taiwanese study.

Remember, this data is still very preliminary. I would predict there will be much more. This "shot gun" nutrient is getting ready to pull the trigger since there are many benefits just waiting to be consumed. Pick the firm ones, with no wrinkles, soft spots, or bruises, and with smooth, deep color. The deeper the color, the better.

God has done everything for us and yet, most times, we choose unwisely. When shopping for your vegetables, look for color, color, color! It's like real estate — location, location, location!

Pumpkin Seeds

These seeds, known as pepitas, are part of the gourd family and come from a yellow-orange vegetable loaded with vitamins, minerals, beta carotene, essential fatty acids, and tryptophan.

1. Have the third highest levels of phytosterols (plant-based estrogen-like chemicals) of seeds and nuts, making them important for breast and prostate problems and their receptor mechanisms. As a matter of fact, in the good saw palmetto preparations, pumpkin seed extract will be added; read the label and look for it.
2. Reduce prostate size and bladder symptoms of having to urinate every thirty minutes, especially at night. One study reported it basically decreases overactive bladder symptoms by 30% in three months.

3. Decrease of lipids of up to 57% and specifically, cholesterol and LDL (bad cholesterol) while raising the HDL (good cholesterol), according to an African study.
4. Shows to be as good as Norvasc in lowering hypertension. I can tell you from personal experience, Norvasc is a good one.
5. May help patients with anxiety and sleep problems because of the tryptophan in it according to a recent Canadian study. Exactly like that huge turkey dinner at Thanksgiving, where everyone after eating it goes to sleep in the living room.

Pumpkin seeds, like stinging nettles, are good add-ons. There will be much more in the future due to their untapped benefits.

Oregano

Another plant that can be grown in your own back yard and is related to the mint family. An herb used a lot in the Mediterranean diet, it loves to grow in pots. The active ingredient, carvacrol, has been shown to:

1. Protect cellular DNA by increasing programmed cell death. The cells do not extend their life spans; an important ingredient for all cancer cells. Prostate cancer cells are a good example.
2. Have anti-inflammatory activity, but the mechanism is still being researched.
3. Have antibacterial activity, which is still very preliminary but surely similar to basil.
4. Can act as a mild diuretic. If you have any fluid retention, herb-up with it. Oregano can be added to many things to enhance the taste.

Sage

Another herb native to the Mediterranean countries, and thus in their diets, has the following chemicals, giving it immense benefit: luteolin, chlorogenic acid, tannic acid, flavones, oleic acid, apigenin, and diosmetin (estrogen like). Once consumed, it is rapidly absorbed and the benefits include:

1. Decreases colon cancer risk because of the apigenin, found in cruciferous vegetables, i.e., broccoli, kale, spinach, etc.
2. Improves cognition, increases attention (ADD-ADHD) accuracy, and improved word recall.
3. Decreases inflammation through luteolin, inhibiting NFkB, TBK1 (TANK binding Kinase), and Cox-2 enzymes.
4. Decreases blood sugar, affecting the insulin resistance.
5. Improves menopausal symptoms, i.e., night sweats, irritability, insomnia, etc.

It's surprising just how many illnesses it can benefit. In 2001, it was voted herb of the year by the International Herb Association.

Cauliflower

Part of the beta-carotene story and the cruciferous family, it has very recently been gaining popularity. Jammed pack with nutrients, it has increased amounts of vitamins C, K, and phytochemicals. The main ones are the glucosinolates that break down into beta isothiocyanate (BITC), and sufurophones along with 13C.

1. BITC has been shown to restore cellular p53, which has an anti-cancer effect. The converse is also true, patients with low levels have an increased cancer risk. The problem resides with a mutation of the DNA that leads to the low levels.
2. Sufurophones induce phase two of our detoxification enzymes that neutralize cancer causing agents. Phase one is only the recognition, but stage two gets rid of it. One serving per week has been shown to decrease lung cancer by 61% and bladder cancer by 27%. Other cancers like esophagus and kidney also see dramatic effects.
3. Decreases cardiovascular deaths by 30%.
4. The increased vitamin C in it reduces inflammation seen in RA.
5. The potassium in it decreases insulin resistance, improving blood sugars in diabetics.

The drum beat of the cruciferous band plays on, but it really depends on who's listening. Listening is not enough since you need them to do the dance of its benefits.

Tomatoes

That red color, yet again, is a billboard to eat tomatoes, and for good reason. The enticing red is due to lycopene, synthesized by the plant's microorganisms. It is part of the carotenoid family and, as with anything fat soluble, it's best to eat them with a meal, letting the fat help with their absorption. We learned, especially with vitamin D, that unless you do this, absorption and blood levels will be low. And, cooking them releases more of the lycopene. Although eating them raw sounds tantalizing, stewing them will give you more nutrition and benefit.

1. Lycopene, a strong antioxidant, targets the prostate. Studies have shown it to help prevent and even treat prostate cancer. For example, eating two-four servings of tomatoes per week was associated with a decrease of prostate cancer by 50%. I generally use it in combination with soy protein, Zyflamend, saw palmetto, EPA oils, green tea, vitamin E, and selenium.

2. May help prevent sun burn through its antioxidant effects of the skin, according to a Harvard study.

3. Rub-on skin preparations have shown it to lessen chronic skin inflammation from the sun and prevent and treat melisma, a dark skin discoloration from the sun.

4. Benefits the retina, according to preliminary studies; no surprise due to its color and the retina's color dependency.

5. Because of its antioxidant activity, it may also prevent other tumors like lung, pancreatic, and breast. Studies have shown low blood levels increase the risk of all three.

6. Inhibits the oxidative damage of LDL (bad cholesterol), and Harvard found eating seven or more servings per week decreased cardiovascular risks by 30%. Then, Finnish researchers found it to decrease carotid artery thickening secondary to atherosclerosis!

Lycopene is just beginning to be understood. The deep red color is its calling card. I not sure if the green and yellow ones would do the same. If you have prostate disease in your family or a Vietnam history with agent-orange expose, you are subject to higher prostate cancer risks, take it as a 15 mg/day established dose. Since there is no risk but great benefit, that ration is where you want it.

Avocados

An ancient fruit whose name is derived from the Aztecs, which means testicles, of all things, because on the tree that's what they look like. For years, it got a bad rap because of the fat in it. But after studying it, we found the fat is monounsaturated, oleic acid, the same found in olive oil, the good kind. With that, some of olive oil's benefits therefore can be transferred over to it. It also has fiber, glutathione, phytosterols, flavonoids and carotenoids, zeaxanthin, and neochrome (a little-known carotenoid).

1. Because of its antioxidants like zeaxanthin, studies have shown it to benefit osteoarthritis, with less pain and swelling and improved cartilage problems.
2. Nuclear cataracts can be reduced by as much as 23%, along with retinal maintenance because of the carotenoid activity. Macular degeneration is a big one, the most common cause of blindness in the U.S. today.
3. It has several mechanisms for cancer prevention, including H. pylori inhibition, which can cause stomach cancer, and it increases glutathione, a long-acting antioxidant to interrupt DNA mutations from inflammation. Even oral lesions can benefit according to recent studies.
4. Because of its excellent supply of fiber and antioxidants, it reduces LDL oxidation, a cause of heart disease, raised cholesterol, and homocysteine levels, all of which prevent atherosclerosis and heart disease. On a three-

week diet of avocados, cholesterol levels decreased 8%.

5. The metabolic syndrome or syndrome "X" has been shown to improve with avocadoes by patients losing weight and lowering lower sugar levels.

6. The carotenoids benefit the skin and avocados are no exception. Studies have shown less wrinkles when consumed, and it is thought secondary to its ability to protect us from the sun's ultraviolet light waves, with lutein and zeaxanthin the major ones.

In summary, avocadoes have a great deal to offer. Again, the drum beat of fiber, antioxidants, and anti-inflammatories are the common denominators. Forget the fat scare; these fats are good, so guacamole-up! We need to forget the old notion of fats being bad because the carbohydrates are the villains.

Garlic

Garlic is a mainstay of the Mediterranean diet, and for good reason; it repels disease. Since it takes twenty minutes to reach its chemical endpoint once the garlic clove is cut (some fourteen chemical steps), wait a bit to cook it (drink some red wine while waiting). We know the most active chemical in it is allicin, but it also contains triterpenoids, flavonoids, glutamyl peptides, Sardinians, and fructans. Dr. Barbara Levine, head of the Garlic Institute at Cornell University, told me garlic is, in fact, excreted through the skin, so if you eat it, others will smell it even after mouth wash. Forget that, it is worth the olfactory overload.

Actions include:

1. Decreases platelet adhesiveness (thus decreasing arteriosclerosis), and prevents heart attacks.
2. Decreases lipids, specifically cholesterol and LDL, the bad cholesterol.
3. Lowers blood pressure (7% systolic and 4% diastolic). In 1996, a study of 1,800 patients over four years showed garlic decreased arterial plaque by 2.6%, and in the placebo group, the plaque increased by 15%.
4. Decreases blood sugar and improves diabetes.
5. Protects from cancer, especially the stomach and bladder.

The dose is brand-directed, but use it in cooking all you can. Indications include: heart disease, elevated lipid levels, general medical care, HBP, diabetes, cancer prevention, and decreased anemia. Don't buy the garlic you see in decorative bottles floating in oil. Garlic can have clostridia botulinum spores on it and, in the no-oxygen environment in the oil, the spores will grow the bacteria, leading to botulism from the toxin they produce.

Berries

This is easy to understand not only because of the color clue, but the variety God has offered us. You can only guess how great they are! What's fascinating is some have different, distinct benefits. The powerful antioxidants and flavonoids are linked and affect most systems and every important disease.

1. Aronia. In animal studies, these berries have a protective effect on the coronary arteries, decrease inflammation of the eye, and inhibit inflammatory markers for colon-cancer cells. It

may have some benefit in improving blood sugar and cholesterol levels as well.

2. Bilberry/Blueberries have been discussed before with their great overall benefit. New data suggests they also improve stomach mucous levels, therefore protecting it from ulcers and H. pylori bacteria.

3. Blackcurrant has mass amounts of vitamin C, even more than oranges. Recent reports show it reduces symptoms of tired eyes, lowers LDL (bad cholesterol) levels, and, in rats, increases life expectance. They dilate blood vessels and have antibacterial actions, which may help urinary-tract infections.

4. Blackberry. Helps with cancer-cell destruction of oral, breast, colon, and prostate cancer cells. It beats out most other antioxidants with a very high ORAC score, directly affecting cardiovascular risk factors.

5. Black Soybean Hull. Through its very strong antioxidant activity, it protects us from the oxidation of lipids. Hardening of the arteries and coronary artery disease are its prime targets.

6. Elderberry. Decreases the virulent effects of the sometimes-fatal influenza virus. Traditionally used during the cold and flu season, it is a good choice. It decreases the damage of free radicals on blood vessels, thus decreasing atherosclerosis.

7. Blue Corn, also known as purple corn, is like yellow corn except it produces a particularly deep purple color and is very potent. Rats fed a diet with this in it had less obesity, diabetes, and suppressed colon-cancer cells. On the ORAC grid for assessing the strength of an antioxidant, it ranks very high, thus making it a great agent in reducing inflammation and all its evil effects.

8. Cherries, sweet or tart, have been shown to be beneficial in reducing inflammation of joints and in the prevention of heart disease. Tart cherries particularly decrease insulin resistance and lower blood sugars by increasing insulin levels. Cancer may also be helped because of perillyl alcohol in them.

I think you get the picture. Berries help a great many things but the trick is to get them into our diets. Make sure you vary the kinds and blend them into a smoothie.

CONCLUSION

This is truly not the final chapter because we are only on the front end of understanding the true benefit of nutrients. As a standard practicing physician with all the essential training, which included nothing on nutrition, I am excited for all of us. We all benefit from their use.

Some things are worth repeating. You must remember, organic turnips will not extend your life unless you do the basics first — diet and exercise. If you want more bang for your buck, and maximum benefit, they need to be an integral part of your life. Health is a team approach — diet, exercise, yearly physical exams to find risk factors and correct them, and nutrients. They *all* need to be done.

Follow the rules of taking nutrients because "more is not better," and don't delude yourself. That's like long-distance runners thinking they are healthier than those doing only moderate exercises three hours weekly.

I underscored important mechanisms like free radicals (oxidation), antioxidants, mitochondria, telomeres, DNA mutations, hormone deficiencies, antioxidant banking, NFkB, and others. These and many more will help guide you through the literature and not be misled by slick marketing techniques to sell you something worthless. This will help you in buying nutrients because you will know what to look for. Since taking nutrients can be burdensome, if you know why you are taking something, you are more likely to do it.

Many times when re-reviewing a manuscript, authors will add updated, newly released data, using phrases such as, "More recently." In reference to nutrition, it concerns mainly the immune system and how it affects cancer, aging, and longevity. I did just that with the information on circulating senescent cells and their effect on inflammation and aging, which will become more prevalent in the news and publications in the near future, and *you* will be on the cutting edge, having read it here first.

Always remember these nutritional recommendations are all done under the permission of your personal physician. Nutrients are chemicals and not innocuous, especially if you are taking other drugs because there can be significant interactions.

My strategy has always been to offer to my patients everything available to improve their life's quality and increase their life spans. Whether it be a magic wand, religion, pet therapy, drugs, surgery, or nutrients, I do it all. Find what works for you, and stick with it, but always be open to improvements and new ideas.

For more information on Dr. Vastola and his practice: Your Good Health www.yourgoodhealthfl.com 1000 Prosperity Farms Rd, Palm Beach Gardens, FL 33410

Issues and their Nutritional Counterparts

Allergies:
        Butterbur, quercetin, vitamin C. My choice: all three.

Alzheimer's disease: See dementia.

Anemia:

    B12, iron, folate. My choice: address whatever it is deficient after testing.

Anxiety:

    Passion flower, ashwagandha, vitamin C, kava, and lavender. My choice: passion flower and lavender.

Arthritis:

    Pomegranate, curry, EPA (fish oil), krill oil, quercetin, borage oil, fax oil, andrographia, UC-11, pycnogenol, glucosamine, MSM, ginger, mung bean extract, and peony extract. My choice: EPA, mung bean extract, peony, glucosamine (for osteoarthritis only), Zyflamend, MSM, ginger, and U.C.-11.

Asthma:

    Butterbur, vitamin C, and quercetin. My choice: all three.

Bladder:

    Arginine, vinpocetine. My choice: vinpocetine.

Bleeding:

    Vitamins K2, vitamin C, vitamin D, and grape seed extract. My choice: grape seed extract and vitamin C; addressing the others with clear deficiencies noted and documented after blood tests.

Balding (men)

    Saw palmetto.

Brain:

Resveratrol, pterostilbene, acetyl-L-carnitine, carnosine, EPA, K2, ashwagandha, lipoic acid, gastrodin, magnesium threonate, taurine, ginseng, arginine, ginkgo, growth hormone, grape seed, vinpocetine, and PS. My choice: gastrodin, magnesium threonate, taurine, vinpocetine, lipoic acid, PS, and ginkgo, and more recently, lithium with proline polypeptide.

Breast:

Soy, maitake, green tea, vitamin D, EPA, 13 C or 3 indole carbinol, and resveratrol. My choice: all of them.

Cancer (depends on primary site i.e. prostate, breast, colon, etc.):

Saw palmetto, lycopene, K2, blueberry, EPA, quercetin, krill oil, CoQ10, PQQ, chlorogenic acid, branched chain amino acids, flax oil, Zyflamend, olive oil, green tea, andrographia, pycnogenols, beta carotene, vitamin B12, ginger, silymarin, garlic, melatonin, pomegranate, selenium, melatonin, turmeric, vitamin E, resveratrol, pterostilbene, vitamin D. My choice: patient would be evaluated, complete histories taken, blood tests analyzed, all physicians consulted along with all medications being taken listed and addressed; would also depend on what we specifically want to prevent or help.

Chronic Fatigue Syndrome:

Ginseng, fucoidans, EPA (omega-3 oils), branched chain amino acids, krill oils, green tea, DHEA, CoQ10, vitamin C and E, lipoic acid, reishi and cistanche, zinc, enzymatic change and rice bran. My choice: reishi, cistanche, rice bran, and ginseng.

Circulation:

Arginine, EPA (omega-3 oils), krill oil, olive oil, pycnogenols, vitamin D, pomegranate, vitamins K2 and E, resveratrol, and pterostilbene. My choice: EPA, vitamin K2, pomegranate, resveratrol/pterostilbene, pycnogenol, and arginine.

Colitis:

Vitamin E, EPA (omega-3 oils), krill oil, B carotene, ginseng, vitamin C, quercetin, folic acid, wheat grass, apple extract, vitamin B12, and probiotic. My choice: EPA, probiotic, wheat grass, apple extract with phloretin, cruciferous extract with apigenin, sulforaphane, and beta isothiocyanate, folic acid, and vitamin B12.

Dementia:

Ginseng, lipoic acid, acetyl-L-carnitine, green tea, gingko, PS, DHEA, vinpocetine, gastrodin, magnesium threonate, taurine, chlorogenic acid, growth hormone, EPA, lithium, and krill oil. My choice: PS, vinpocetine, gastrodin, magnesium threonate, acetyl-L-carnitine, lithium, green tea, taurine, and gingko.

Depression:

St. John's Wort (early and on no other medication), EPA (omega-3 oils), SAM-e, and pregnenolone. My choice: St. John's Wort and SAM-e.

Diabetes mellitus:

Turmeric, carnosine, branched chains amino acids, chlorogenic acid, fucoidans, lipoic acid, chromium, pomegranate, EPA (omega-3 and 7 oils), krill oil, olive oil, green tea, pycnogenols, DHEA, CoQ10, PQQ, garlic, soy, resveratrol, blueberry, red yeast rice. My choice: blueberry (bilberry), chlorogenic acid, chromium, carnosine, resveratrol, turmeric, AMPK, and omega 3 and 7 oils.

Eye:
Lutein, zeaxanthin, blueberry, marine bark (pycnogenol), carnosine, EPA, krill, beta carotene, vitamin C, lycopene. My choice: all but krill oil.

General Medical Care:
Pterostilbene, resveratrol, vitamin B3, vitamin D, CoQ10, PQQ, carnitine, branched chain amino acids, pomegranate, EPA (omega-3 oils), carnosine, olive oil, green tea, pycnogenol, beta carotene, growth hormone, DHEA, lipoic acid, blueberry, vitamin K2, garlic, quercetin, turmeric, and selenium with vitamin E. My choice: incorporate the patient's medical condition, prevailing problems, and current medications. There is no set template. Everyone is unique, requiring each prescription, whether for nutrients, supplements, or prescription meds, to be customized.

Hair loss (men):
Saw palmetto.

Hair loss (women):
Grape seed extract.

Heart:
Quercetin, turmeric, vitamin K2, carnitine, pomegranate, carnosine, EPA (omega-3 oils), krill oil, branched chain amino acids, acetyl-L-carnitine, CoQ10, PQQ, green tea, pycnogenol, olive oil, lipoic acid, vitamin D, growth hormone, blueberry, red yeast rice, hawthorne, garlic, vitamin E, selenium, resveratrol, and pterostilbene. My choice: dependent on underlying problems and co-morbidities, like HBP, elevated lipids,

etc. Must be determined after a complete medical exam and research of what is being taken, whether it is nutrients, supplements, or prescription meds. Many things may be contraindicated. Basic formula would include carnitine, lipoic acid, branched chain amino acids, taurine, and CoQ10/PQQ

Hypertension (HBP):

Pomegranate, resveratrol, passion flower, olive oil, green tea, pycnogenol, hawthorne, garlic, taurine, and CoQ10. My choice: Hawthorne, CoQ10/PQQ, taurine, and olive oil.

Immunity:

Ginseng, EPA, krill oil, selenium, beta carotene, flax oil, vitamin E, pycnogenol, quercetin, growth hormone, DHEA, reishi, cistanche, zinc, enzymatic converted rice bran, fucoidans, branched chain amino acids, and probiotic. My choice: probiotic, beta carotene, selenium, vitamins C and E, reishi, cistanche, zinc, and fucoidans.

Irritable bowel syndrome (IBS):

Probiotic, peppermint.

Jet lag:

Melatonin.

Leukemia:

Vitamin K2, ginger, turmeric, resveratrol, and zinc.

Libido:

DHEA, pomegranate and pregnenolone.

Lipids:

Red yeast rice, guggal, policosanol, vitamin K2, pomegranate, turmeric, olive oil, EPA (omega-3 and 7 oils), and garlic. My choice: red rice yeast, guggal, olive oil, and EPA.

Liver:
Silymarin.

Lungs:
Growth hormone, cysteine with glutathione, and green tea. My choice: cysteine/glutathione.

Lupus erythematosus:
DHEA, green tea, mung bean extract, 3 indole carbinol (13C), zinc, and peony extract. My choice: all of them, and they work!

Menopause:
See PMS.

Migraine:
Butterbur and feverfew. My choice: butterbur.

Muscle problems:
Carnitine, carnosine, B carotene, chromium, ginseng, pregnenolone, branched chain amino acid, growth hormone, CoQ10, PQQ, and lipoic acid. My choice: carnitine, carnosine, CoQ10, PQQ, branched chain amino acids, and lipoic acid.

Nails:
Grape seed extract. My choice: since it works, but you need to be patient — one to two months to work. Nails grow v-e-r-y s-l-o-w-l-y.

Neuropathy:

Pycnogenol, B12, Huperzine, vinpocetine, vitamin B complex, and lipoic acid. My choice: Huperzine, vitamin B complex, vinpocetine, pycnogenol, and lipoic acid. In my experience, they work better than standard expensive medication with fewer side effects. You need to be patient since nerves grow very slowly. You are looking at two-three months for the symptoms to diminish before there is improvement.

Obesity:

White bean extract, Irvingia, and l-arabinose inhibitor. My choice: Irvingia and, again, you must be patient. Exercise and calorie restrict yourself, otherwise it won't work. Let me comment on the diet thing since there is an abundance of misinformation out there to confuse you. The best diet is the Adkins's diet since it restricts carbohydrates, the bad guys. Not only will your weight come down over an extended period, but your blood parameters will improve, like your blood sugar, lipids, etc. Numerous studies prove these statements, but in addition, there is evidence this diet helps in preventing cancer, the number-two killer of Americans today, by preventing the insulin surge with meals. Insulin is a tissue growth factor. My next choice once you reach the ideal weight (BMI between 25-30) would be the Mediterranean diet.

Osteoporosis:

Carnitine, growth hormone, olive oil, strontium, boron, DHEA, vitamin K2, lycopene, vitamin D3, soy, and calcium. For premenopausal women, 1200 mg of calcium is necessary with vitamin D3, and for postmenopausal women, 1500 mg is necessary. Make sure the calcium is not the calcium carbonate since only 20% is absorbed. Any other calcium preparation is adequate, like calcium sulfate. If your DEXA scan, the test done for osteoporosis, is positive for osteoporosis, then a medication like Fosamax should also be added. My choice: calcium, vitamin D3 (5000 i.u./day), strontium, boron, and the medication if indicated.

Parkinsonism:
Lipoic acid, CoQ10/PQQ, vitamin D3, and PQQ. My choice: All three, but the dose of CoQ10 needs to be 900-1200 mg/day. Make sure the CoQ10 is ubiquinol, not ubiquinone; the former is much better absorbed.

PMS (premenstrual syndrome) and Menopause:
Flax seed oil, black cohosh, green tea, EPA (omega-3 oils), and soy. My choice: soy, green tea, and black cohosh together.

Prostate disease:
Soy protein, lycopene, saw palmetto, selenium with vitamin E, beta sitosterol, EPA (omega-3 oils), maitake, green tea, and Zyflamend. My choices: are all of them together for BPH (benign prostatic hypertrophy) or cancer, with the exception of maitake.

Let me share a true story regarding one of my patients. I realize it represents anecdote, but this shared experience may reinforce these supplements concerning a case of prostate disease. This fifty-four-year-old male patient was diagnosed with cancer of the prostate with a very high Glisson score; an indication of its malignancy. He refused the standard medical therapy of surgery and postop radiation because he "just didn't want it." When he came to me, I advised strongly for him to go with the standard therapies, but again he refused, knowing full well supplements might not help and would delay further his needed care. Within three months, his PSA came down from fifteen to five, and a repeat biopsy of the prostate was negative for cancer. His urologist was astounded, and even more befuddled, when he found out why, refusing to accept it. To this day, seven years later, he is cancer-free with repeat biopsies and a PSA level of five. Now this heroic story of one does not set precedent, but I think there is some merit in its telling.

Raynaud's disease:

Arginine, peony extract, 13C (3 indole carbinol), and mung bean extract. My choice: all four.

Skin problems-bleeding:

Grape seed extract, vitamin C, lycopene.

Sleep problems:

Kava, valerian, melatonin, passion flower, ashwagandha, and lavender. My choice: combination of melatonin and lavender. One warning: the melatonin will be a miracle with sleep or not work at all. There will be no in-between.

Stomach and GERD or (reflux):

Olive oil, green tea, vitamin B-12, ginger, turmeric, licorice DGL (deglycyrrhizinated licorice), peppermint, and probiotic. My choice: green tea, olive oil, and DGL. More recently, zinc, 75 mg with Lactobacillus reuteri.

Tinnitus (ringing in ears):

Vinpocetine.

Urinary tract infections (UTI):

Cranberry extract and probiotic.

Vaginosis:

Probiotics.

Viruses:

Echinacea, andrographia, zinc, DHEA, vitamins C and D, panax in ginseng, reishi, cistanche, enzymatic changed rice bran, fucoidans, branched chain amino acids, and beta carotene. My choice: really depends on the clinical situation and the strain of virus.

BIBLIOGRAPHY

Abuelgassim, Ao, and Sia Al-Showayman. "The Effect of Pumpkin (*Cucurbita Pepo* L) Seeds and L-Arginine Supplementation on Serum Lipid Concentrations in Atherogenic Rats." *African Journal of Traditional, Complementary and Alternative Medicines Afr. J. Trad. Compl. Alt. Med.* 9, no. 1 (2011). doi:10.4314/ajtcam.v9i1.18.

Adebamowo, Clement A., Eunyoung Cho, Laura Sampson, Martijn B. Katan, Donna Spiegelman, Walter C. Willett, and Michelle D. Holmes. "Dietary Flavanols and Flavanol-rich Foods Intake and the Risk of Breast Cancer." *International Journal of Cancer Int. J. Cancer* 114, no. 4 (2005): 628-33. doi:10.1002/ijc.20741.

McLendon. "African Mango (Irvingia Gabonensis) Extract for Weight Loss: A Systematic Review." *Journal of Nutritional Therapeutics J. Nutr. Ther.*, 2013. doi:10.6000/1929-5634.2013.02.01.7.
Ames, Bruce. "Free Radicals." *Discover Magazine*, October 1, 2002.

Ames, Bruce N., and Jiankang Liu. "Delaying the Mitochondrial Decay of Aging with Acetyl-L-Carnitine." *Annals of the New York Academy of Sciences* 1033, no. 1 (2004): 108-16. doi:10.1196/annals.1320.010.

Arendash, Cao. "Caffeine and Coffee as

Therapeutic against Alzheimer's Disease." *Journal of Alzheimer's Disease* 20, no. 1 (2010): 117-26.

Aviram, Michael, and Leslie Dornfeld. "Pomegranate Juice Consumption Inhibits Serum Angiotensin Converting Enzyme Activity and Reduces Systolic Blood Pressure." *Atherosclerosis* 158, no. 1 (2001): 195-98. doi:10.1016/s0021-9150(01)00412-9.

Aviram, Michael, and Mira Rosenblatt. "Pomegranate for Your Cardiovascular Health." *RMMJ Rambam Maimonides Medical Journal* 4, no. 2 (2013). doi:10.5041/rmmj.10113.

Bagchi, D., A. Garg, R.L. Krohn, M. Bagchi, D.J. Bagchi, J. Balmoori, and S.J. Stohs. "Protective Effects of Grape Seed Proanthocyanidins and Selected Antioxidants against TPA-Induced Hepatic and Brain Lipid Peroxidation and DNA Fragmentation, and Peritoneal Macrophage Activation in Mice." *General Pharmacology: The Vascular System* 30, no. 5 (1998): 771-76. doi:10.1016/s0306-3623(97)00332-7.

Baker, Michael E. "Licorice and Enzymes Other than 11β-hydroxysteroid Dehydrogenase: An Evolutionary Perspective." *Steroids* 59, no. 2 (1994): 136-41. doi:10.1016/0039-128x(94)90091-4.

Bar-Sela, Gil, Medy Tsalic, Getta Fried, and Hadassah Goldberg. "Wheat Grass Juice May Improve Hematological Toxicity Related to

Chemotherapy in Breast Cancer Patients: A Pilot Study." *Nutrition and Cancer* 58, no. 1 (2007): 43-48. doi:10.1080/01635580701308083.

Barve, Avantika, Tin Oo Khor, Sujit Nair, Kenneth Reuhl, Nanjoo Suh, Bandaru Reddy, Harold Newmark, and Ah-Ng Kong. "γ-Tocopherol-enriched Mixed Tocopherol Diet Inhibits Prostate Carcinogenesis in TRAMP Mice." *International Journal of Cancer Int. J. Cancer* 124, no. 7 (2009): 1693-699. doi:10.1002/ijc.24106.

Becker, David J., Benjamin French, Patti B. Morris, Erin Silvent, and Ram Y. Gordon. "Phytosterols, Red Yeast Rice, and Lifestyle Changes Instead of Statins: A Randomized, Double-blinded, Placebo-controlled Trial." *American Heart Journal* 166, no. 1 (2013). doi:10.1016/j.ahj.2013.03.019.

Ben-Arye, E., E. Goldin, D. Wengrower, A. Stamper, R. Kohn, and E. Berry. "Wheat Grass Juice in the Treatment of Active Distal Ulcerative Colitis: A Randomized Double-blind Placebo-controlled Trial." *Scandinavian Journal of Gastroenterology* 37, no. 4 (2002): 444-49. doi:10.1080/003655202317316088.

Berges, R.R., A. Kassen, and T. Senge. "Treatment of Symptomatic Benign Prostatic Hyperplasia with β-sitosterol: An Eighteen-month Follow-up." *BJU International* 85, no. 7 (2001): 842-46. doi:10.1046/j.1464-410x.2000.00672.x.

Beulens, Joline W.J., Michiel L. Bots, Femke Atsma, Marie-Louise E.L. Bartelink, Matthias Prokop, Johanna M. Geleijnse, Jacqueline C.M. Witteman, Diederick E. Grobbee, and Yvonne T. Van Der Schouw. "High Dietary Menaquinone Intake Is Associated with Reduced Coronary Calcification." *Atherosclerosis* 203, no. 2 (2009): 489-93. doi:10.1016/j.atherosclerosis.2008.07.010.

Boerner, R.J., H. Sommer, W. Berger, U. Kuhn, U. Schmidt, and M. Mannel. "Kava-Kava Extract LI 150 Is as Effective as Opipramol and Buspirone in Generalized Anxiety Disorder – An Eight-week Randomized, Double-blind Multi-centre Clinical Trial in 129 Out-patients." *Phytomedicine* 10 (2003): 38-49. doi:10.1078/1433-187x-00309.

Budoff, M. "Inhibiting Progression of Coronary Calcification Using Aged Garlic Extract in Patients Receiving Statin Therapy: A Preliminary Study*1." *Preventive Medicine* 39, no. 5 (2004): 985-91. doi:10.1016/j.ypmed.2004.04.012.

Budoff, Matthew J., Naser Ahmadi, Khawar M. Gul, Sandy T. Liu, Ferdinand R. Flores, Jima Tiano, Junichiro Takasu, Elizabeth Miller, and Sotirios Tsimikas. "Aged Garlic Extract Supplemented with B Vitamins, Folic Acid and L-arginine Retards the Progression of Subclinical Atherosclerosis: A Randomized Clinical Trial." *Preventive Medicine* 49, no. 2-3 (2009): 101-07. doi:10.1016/j.ypmed.2009.06.018.

Cannell, John. "Why Does Vitamin D Council Recommend 5,000 i.u./day." *Vitamin Council Newsletter*, December 10, 2013.

Carr, Anitra, and Balz Frei. "The Role of Natural Antioxidants in Preserving the Biological Activity of Endothelium-derived Nitric Oxide." *Free Radical Biology and Medicine* 28, no. 12 (2000): 1806-814. doi:10.1016/s0891-5849(00)00225-2.

Cerhan. "Mayo Clinic Study Links Increased Vitamin K Intake to Lower Non-Hodgkin's Lymphoma Risk." *Featured Article in Life Extension and Journal of Cancer*, April 27, 2010.

Cesarone, M. R., G. Belcaro, S. Stuard, F. Schonlau, A. Di Renzo, M. G. Grossi, M. Dugall, U. Cornelli, M. Cacchio, G. Gizzi, and L. Pellegrini. "Kidney Flow and Function in Hypertension: Protective Effects of Pycnogenol in Hypertensive Participants--A Controlled Study." *Journal of Cardiovascular Pharmacology and Therapeutics* 15, no. 1 (2010): 41-46. doi:10.1177/1074248409356063.

Chang, Hui-Hsin, Kuang-Yang Hsieh, Chen-Hao Yeh, Yuan-Ping Tu, and Fuu Sheu. "Oral Administration of an Enoki Mushroom Protein FVE Activates Innate and Adaptive Immunity and Induces Anti-tumor Activity against Murine Hepatocellular Carcinoma." *International Immunopharmacology* 10, no. 2 (2010): 239-46. doi:10.1016/j.intimp.2009.10.017.

Chang, Jaewon, Agnes Rimando, Merce Pallas, Antoni Camins, David Porquet, Jennifer Reeves, Barbara Shukitt-Hale, Mark A. Smith, James A. Joseph, and Gemma Casadesus. "Low-dose Pterostilbene, but Not Resveratrol, Is a Potent Neuromodulator in Aging and Alzheimer's Disease." *Neurobiology of Aging* 33, no. 9 (2012): 2062-071. doi:10.1016/j.neurobiolaging.2011.08.015.

Cholujova, Dana, Jana Jakubikova, Branislav Czako, Michaela Martisova, Luba Hunakova, Jozef Duraj, Martin Mistrik, and Jan Sedlak. "MGN-3 Arabinoxylan Rice Bran Modulates Innate Immunity in Multiple Myeloma Patients." *Cancer Immunology, Immunotherapy Cancer Immunol Immunother* 62, no. 3 (2012): 437-45. doi:10.1007/s00262-012-1344-z.

Chung, I.-M., M.-A. Yeo, S.-J. Kim, and H.-I. Moon. "Protective Effects of Organic Solvent Fractions from the Seeds of Vigna Radiata L. Wilczek against Antioxidant Mechanisms." *Human & Experimental Toxicology* 30, no. 8 (2010): 904-09. doi:10.1177/0960327110382565.

Clark, L. C. "Effects of Selenium Supplementation for Cancer Prevention in Patients with Carcinoma of the Skin. A Randomized Controlled Trial. Nutritional Prevention of Cancer Study Group." *JAMA: The Journal of the American Medical Association* 276, no. 24 (1996): 1957-963. doi:10.1001/jama.276.24.1957.

Clark, L. C. "Effects of Selenium Supplementation for Cancer Prevention in Patients with Carcinoma of the Skin. A Randomized Controlled Trial. Nutritional Prevention of Cancer Study Group." *JAMA: The Journal of the American Medical Association* 276, no. 24 (1996): 1957-963. doi:10.1001/jama.276.24.1957.

Clinic, Mayo. "Strong Evidence Supports the Use of Glucosamine Sulfate Taken by Mouth to Treat Osteoarthritis 1998-2016." *Mayo Clinic Review*, November 2013.

Crowley, David C. "Safety and Efficacy of Undenatured Type II Collagen in the Treatment of Osteoarthritis of the Knee: A Clinical Trial." *International Journal of Medical Sciences Int. J. Med. Sci.*, 2009, 312. doi:10.7150/ijms.6.312.
Dreher, Mark L., and Adrienne J. Davenport. "Hass Avocado Composition and Potential Health Effects." *Critical Reviews in Food Science and Nutrition* 53, no. 7 (2013): 738-50. doi:10.1080/10408398.2011.556759.

Eagleton, Morris. "Turn off the Cytokine Switch." *Life Extension Magazine*, January 2014.

"Experimental Animal Laboratory. Final Report for Study on CCO Oil on the Development of Atherosclerosis." *Department of Cardiovascular Medicine, Cleveland Clinic,* 2008.

Fitzpatrick, David F., Bettye Bing, and Peter

Rohdewald. "Endothelium-Dependent Vascular Effects of Pycnogenol." *Journal of Cardiovascular Pharmacology* 32, no. 4 (1998): 509-15. doi:10.1097/00005344-199810000-00001.

Freedman, Neal D., Yikyung Park, Christian C. Abnet, Albert R. Hollenbeck, and Rashmi Sinha. "Association of Coffee Drinking with Total and Cause-Specific Mortality." *New England Journal of Medicine N Engl J Med* 366, no. 20 (2012): 1891-904. doi:10.1056/nejmoa1112010.

Fulgoni, Victor L., Mark Dreher, and Adrienne J. Davenport. "Avocado Consumption Is Associated with Better Diet Quality and Nutrient Intake, and Lower Metabolic Syndrome Risk in U.S. Adults: Results from the National Health and Nutrition Examination Survey (NHANES) 2001–2008." *Nutrition Journal Nutr J* 12, no. 1 (2013). doi:10.1186/1475-2891-12-1.

Gebara, Elias, Florian Udry, Sébastien Sultan, and Nicolas Toni. "Taurine Increases Hippocampal Neurogenesis in Aging Mice." *Stem Cell Research* 14, no. 3 (2015): 369-79. doi:10.1016/j.scr.2015.04.001.

Ghanim, Husam, Chang Ling Sia, Sanaa Abuaysheh, Kelly Korzeniewski, Priyanka Patnaik, Anuritha Marumganti, Ajay Chaudhuri, and Paresh Dandona. "An Anti-inflammatory and Reactive Oxygen Species Suppressive Effects of an Extract of Polygonum Cuspidatum

Containing Resveratrol." *Molecular Endocrinology* 24, no. 7 (2010): 1498-499. doi:10.1210/mend.24.7.9998.

Ghoneum, Mamdooh, and Sarah Abedi. "Enhancement of Natural Killer Cell Activity of Aged Mice by Modified Arabinoxylan Rice Bran (MGN-3/Biobran)." *Journal of Pharmacy and Pharmacology* 56, no. 12 (2004): 1581-588. doi:10.1211/0022357044922.

Giovannucci, Edward. "Expanding Role of Vitamin D." *Journal Clinical Endocrinology Metabolism* 94 (2009): 418-20.

Greenberg, James A., Sara J. Newmann, and Amy B. Howell. "Consumption of Sweetened Dried Cranberries Versus Unsweetened Raisins for Inhibition of Uropathogenic Escherichia Coli Adhesion in Human Urine: A Pilot Study." *The Journal of Alternative and Complementary Medicine* 11, no. 5 (2005): 875-78. doi:10.1089/acm.2005.11.875.

Grigoleit, H.-G., and P. Grigoleit. "Peppermint Oil in Irritable Bowel Syndrome." *Phytomedicine* 12, no. 8 (2005): 601-06. doi:10.1016/j.phymed.2004.10.005.

Habs, M. "Prospective, Comparative Cohort Studies and Their Contribution to the Benefit Assessments of Therapeutic Options: Heart Failure Treatment with and without Hawthorn Special Extract WS® 1442." *Forsch Komplementmed Forschende Komplementärmedizin / Research in*

Complementary Medicine 11, no. 1 (2004): 36-39. doi:10.1159/000080574.

Hardman, Elaine. "How Omega 3 Fats May Protect Against Cancer." *American Institute for Cancer Research Newsletter, Pennington Bio Med Research Center, LSU* 84 (June/July 2004). Hardman, W. E. "Breast Cancer Risk Drops When Diet Includes Walnuts." *Nutrition and Cancer- Marshall University Research Group*, September 1, 2011.

Harper, C. E., B. B. Patel, J. Wang, A. Arabshahi, I. A. Eltoum, and C. A. Lamartiniere. "Resveratrol Suppresses Prostate Cancer Progression in Transgenic Mice." *Carcinogenesis* 28, no. 9 (2007): 1946-953. doi:10.1093/carcin/bgm144.

Harris, Calliandra B., Winyoo Chowanadisai, Darya O. Mishchuk, Mike A. Satre, Carolyn M. Slupsky, and Robert B. Rucker. "Dietary Pyrroloquinoline Quinone (PQQ) Alters Indicators of Inflammation and Mitochondrial-related Metabolism in Human Subjects." *The Journal of Nutritional Biochemistry* 24, no. 12 (2013): 2076-084. doi:10.1016/j.jnutbio.2013.07.008j.

Hartman, Johan, Anders Ström, and Jan-Åke Gustafsson. "Estrogen Receptor Beta in Breast Cancer — Diagnostic and Therapeutic Implications." *Steroids* 74, no. 8 (2009): 635-41. doi:10.1016/j.steroids.2009.02.005.

He, Ka. "Fish, Long-Chain Omega-3

Polyunsaturated Fatty Acids and Prevention of Cardiovascular Disease — Eat Fish or Take Fish Oil Supplement?" *Progress in Cardiovascular Diseases* 52, no. 2 (2009): 95-114. doi:10.1016/j.pcad.2009.06.003.

Heuser, Gunnar, and Aristo Vojdani. "Enhancement of Natural Killer Cell Activity and T and B Cell Function by Buffered Vitamin C in Patients Exposed to Toxic Chemicals: The Role of Protein Kinase-C." *Immunopharmacology and Immunotoxicology* 19, no. 3 (1997): 291-312. doi:10.3109/08923979709046977.

Hipkiss, Alan R., and Harj Chana. "Carnosine Protects Proteins against Methylglyoxal-Mediated Modifications." *Biochemical and Biophysical Research Communications* 248, no. 1 (1998): 28-32. doi:10.1006/bbrc.1998.8806.

Ho, Yi-Jin, Wen-Pin Chen, Tzong-Cherng Chi, Ching-Chia Chang Chien, An-Sheng Lee, Hsi-Lin Chiu, Yueh-Hsiung Kuo, and Ming-Jai Su. "Caffeic Acid Phenethyl Amide Improves Glucose Homeostasis and Attenuates the Progression of Vascular Dysfunction in Streptozotocin-induced Diabetic Rats." *Cardiovasc Diabetol Cardiovascular Diabetology* 12, no. 1 (2013): 99. doi:10.1186/1475-2840-12-99.

Hsu, Anna, Richard S. Bruno, Christiane V. Löhr, Alan W. Taylor, Rodrick H. Dashwood, Tammy M. Bray, and Emily Ho. "Dietary Soy and Tea Mitigate Chronic Inflammation and

Prostate Cancer via NFkB Pathway in the Noble Rat Model." *The Journal of Nutritional Biochemistry* 22, no. 5 (2011): 502-10. doi:10.1016/j.jnutbio.2010.04.006.

Hsu, Guoo-Shyng Wang, Yi-Fa Lu, Shu-Hwa Chang, and Shun-Yao Hsu. "Antihypertensive Effect of Mung Bean Sprout Extracts in Spontaneously Hypertensive Rats." *Journal of Food Biochemistry* 35, no. 1 (2011): 278-88. doi:10.1111/j.1745-4514.2010.00381.x.

Hulme, A. C. "The Isolation of Chlorogenic Acid from the Apple Fruit." *Biochem. J. Biochemical Journal* 53, no. 3 (1953): 337-40. doi:10.1042/bj0530337.

Hume, Anne L. "Zyflamend for Prevention of Prostate Cancer: Studies Show Benefits, but Larger Trials Needed." *Pharmacy Today* 20, no. 7 (2014): 30. doi:10.1016/s1042-0991(15)30779-9.

Jancin, Bruce. "Flaxseed Supplements Curbed Hot Flashes in Study." *Ob.Gyn. News* 40, no. 3 (2005): 18. doi:10.1016/s0029-7437(05)70793-x.

Kato, Ikuko, Suketami Tominaga, Akira Matsuura, Yuri Yoshii, Masato Shirai, and Seibi Kobayashi. "A Comparative Case-Control Study of Colorectal Cancer and Adenoma." *Japanese Journal of Cancer Research* 81, no. 11 (1990): 1101-108. doi:10.1111/j.1349-7006.1990.tb02520.x.

Kelly, G.S. "A Review of the Sirtuin System, Its Clinical Implications and Potential Role of Dietary Activators like Resveratrol." *Alternative Med Rev*, 2nd ser., 15, no. 4 (December 2010): 313-28.

Kerksick, Chad, and Darryn Willoughby. "The Antioxidant Role of Glutathione and N-Acetyl-Cysteine Supplements and Exercise-Induced Oxidative Stress." *J Int Soc Sports Nutr Journal of the International Society of Sports Nutrition* 2, no. 2 (2005): 38. doi:10.1186/1550-2783-2-2-38.

Koz, Sema T., Giyasettin Baydas, Suleyman Koz, Nevgul Demir, and Viktor S. Nedzvetsky. "Gingko Biloba Extract Inhibits Oxidative Stress and Ameliorates Impaired Glial Fibrillary Acidic Protein Expression, but Can Not Improve Spatial Learning in Offspring from Hyperhomocysteinemic Rat Dams." *Phytother. Res. Phytotherapy Research* 26, no. 7 (2011): 949-55. doi:10.1002/ptr.3669.

Langsjoen, Peter H., and Alena M. Langsjoen. "Overview of the Use of CoQ10 in Cardiovascular Disease." *BioFactors* 9, no. 2-4 (1999): 273-84. doi:10.1002/biof.5520090224.
Lehmann, Konrad, André Steinecke, and Jürgen Bolz. "GABA through the Ages: Regulation of Cortical Function and Plasticity by Inhibitory Interneurons." *Neural Plasticity* 2012 (2012): 1-11. doi:10.1155/2012/892784.

Liang, Ji-Yong, Yi-Yan Liu, Jing Zou, Renty B. Franklin, Leslie C. Costello, and Pei Feng.

"Inhibitory Effect of Zinc on Human Prostatic Carcinoma Cell Growth." *The Prostate Prostate* 40, no. 3 (1999): 200-07. doi:10.1002/(sici)1097-0045(19990801)40:33.0.co;2-3.

Lipton, R. B., H. Gobel, K. M. Einhaupl, K. Wilks, and A. Mauskop. "Petasites Hybridus Root (butterbur) Is an Effective Preventive Treatment for Migraine." *Neurology* 63, no. 12 (2004): 2240-244. doi:10.1212/01.wnl.0000147290.68260.11.

Lissoni, P., S. Barni, S. Crispino, G. Tancini, and F. Fraschini. "Endocrine and Immune Effects of Melatonin Therapy in Metastatic Cancer Patients." *European Journal of Cancer and Clinical Oncology* 25, no. 5 (1989): 789-95. doi:10.1016/0277-5379(89)90122-3.

Lissoni, P., M. Chilelli, S. Villa, L. Cerizza, and G. Tancini. "Five Years Survival in Metastatic Non-small Cell Lung Cancer Patients Treated with Chemotherapy Alone or Chemotherapy and Melatonin: A Randomized Trial." *J Pineal Res Journal of Pineal Research* 35, no. 1 (2003): 12-15. doi:10.1034/j.1600-079x.2003.00032.x.

Liu, Jun, Zheng-Tao Wang, Li-Li Ji, and Bao-Xue Ge. "Inhibitory Effects of Neoandrographolide on Nitric Oxide and Prostaglandin E2 Production in LPS-stimulated Murine Macrophage." *Molecular and Cellular Biochemistry Mol Cell Biochem* 298, no. 1-2 (2006): 49-57. doi:10.1007/s11010-006-9349-6.

"Lycopene: What is Its Benefits, How to Increase in Diet," *Harvard News Letter (www.bhia.org)*, 1995.

Ma, Y., V. Y. Njike, J. Millet, S. Dutta, K. Doughty, J. A. Treu, and D. L. Katz. "Effects of Walnut Consumption on Endothelial Function in Type 2 Diabetic Subjects: A Randomized Controlled Crossover Trial." *Diabetes Care* 33, no. 2 (2009): 227-32. doi:10.2337/dc09-1156.
Macdonald, John F., Michael F. Jackson, and Michael A. Beazely. "Hippocampal Long-Term Synaptic Plasticity and Signal Amplification of NMDA Receptors." *Crit Rev Neurobiol Critical Reviews™ in Neurobiology* 18, no. 1-2 (2006): 71-84. doi:10.1615/critrevneurobiol.v18.i1-2.80.

Maher, Diane M., Maria C. Bell, Emmylu A. O'Donnell, Brij K. Gupta, Meena Jaggi, and Subhash C. Chauhan. "Curcumin Suppresses Human Papillomavirus Oncoproteins, Restores P53, Rb, and Ptpn13 Proteins and Inhibits Benzopyrene-induced Upregulation of HPV E7." *Mol. Carcinog. Molecular Carcinogenesis* 50, no. 1 (2010): 47-57. doi:10.1002/mc.20695.
Maheshwari, Radha K., Anoop K. Singh, Jaya Gaddipati, and Rikhab C. Srimal. "Multiple Biological Activities of Curcumin: A Short Review." *Life Sciences* 78, no. 18 (2006): 2081-087. doi:10.1016/j.lfs.2005.12.007.

Maruyama, Hiroko, Hidekazu Tamauchi, Mariko Iizuka, and Takahisa Nakano. "The Role of NK Cells in Anti-tumor Activity of Dietary Fucoidan from Undaria Pinnatifida

Sporophylls (Mekabu)." *Planta Med Planta Medica* 72, no. 15 (2006): 1415-417. doi:10.1055/s-2006-951703.

McGowan. "Epigenics and Mood Disorders." *Environmental Health Med* 13, no. 1 (January 2008): 16-24.

Medjakovic, Svjetlana, Stefanie Hobiger, Karin Ardjomand-Woelkart, Franz Bucar, and Alois Jungbauer. "Pumpkin Seed Extract: Cell Growth Inhibition of Hyperplastic and Cancer Cells, Independent of Steroid Hormone Receptors." *Fitoterapia* 110 (2016): 150-56. doi:10.1016/j.fitote.2016.03.010.

Micheletti, R., G. Giacalone, and G. Bianchi. "Effect of Propionyl-L-Carnitine on the Mechanics of Right and Left Papillary Muscles from Volume-Overloaded Rat Hearts." *Journal of Cardiovascular Pharmacology* 27, no. 1 (1996): 52-57. doi:10.1097/00005344-199601000-00009.

Min, Y.-D., C.-H. Choi, H. Bark, H.-Y. Son, H.-H. Park, S. Lee, J.-W. Park, E.-K. Park, H.-I. Shin, and S.-H. Kim. "Quercetin Inhibits Expression of Inflammatory Cytokines through Attenuation of NF-κB and P38 MAPK in HMC-1 Human Mast Cell Line." *Inflamm. Res. Inflammation Research* 56, no. 5 (2007): 210-15. doi:10.1007/s00011-007-6172-9.

Min, Y.-D., C.-H. Choi, H. Bark, H.-Y. Son, H.-H. Park, S. Lee, J.-W. Park, E.-K. Park, H.-I. Shin, and S.-H. Kim. "Quercetin Inhibits

Expression of Inflammatory Cytokines through Attenuation of NF-κB and P38 MAPK in HMC-1 Human Mast Cell Line." *Inflamm. Res. Inflammation Research* 56, no. 5 (2007): 210-15. doi:10.1007/s00011-007-6172-9.

Moncada, Salvador, Richard M.J. Palmer, and E. Annie Higgs. "Biosynthesis of Nitric Oxide from L-arginine." *Biochemical Pharmacology* 38, no. 11 (1989): 1709-715. doi:10.1016/0006-2952(89)90403-6.

Moore, Amber. "Broccoli Compound Kills Cancer Cells." *Science/technology (PlosOne) Sloan Kettering Cancer Institute*, December 13, 2012.

Murphy JJ, Heptinstall S, Mitchell JR. "Randomized Double-blind Placebo-controlled Trial of Feverfew in Migraine Prevention." *Complementary Therapies in Medicine* 6, no. 2 (1998): 106. doi:10.1016/s0965-2299(98)80095-2.

Müller, Walter E., Anne Eckert, Christopher Kurz, Gunter Peter Eckert, and Kristina Leuner. "Mitochondrial Dysfunction: Common Final Pathway in Brain Aging and Alzheimer's Disease-Therapeutic Aspects." *Molecular Neurobiology Mol Neurobiol* 41, no. 2-3 (2010): 159-71. doi:10.1007/s12035-010-8141-5.

Münch, Gerald, Samantha Mayer, Jürgen Michaelis, Alan R. Hipkiss, Peter Riederer, Renate Müller, Arne Neumann, Reinhard Schinzel, and Anne M. Cunningham. "Influence of Advanced Glycation End-products and AGE-inhibitors on Nucleation-dependent Polymerization of β-amyloid Peptide." *Biochimica Et Biophysica Acta (BBA) - Molecular Basis of Disease* 1360, no. 1 (1997): 17-29. doi:10.1016/s0925-4439(96)00062-2.

Noda, Yasuko, Akitane Mori, Lester Packer, Kazunori Anzai, Masahiro Kohno, and Masashi Shinmei. "Hydroxyl and Superoxide Anion Radical Scavenging Activities of Natural Source Antioxidants Using the Computerized JES-FR30 ESR Spectrometer System." *IUBMB Life TBMB* 42, no. 1 (1997): 35-44. doi:10.1080/15216549700202411.

Oladunmoye M. Kolawole. "Comparative Studies on the Antimicrobial Activity of Leaf Extract from Ocimum Basilicum and Antagonistic Activity of Isolates from Refuse on Some Selected Pathogens." *International Journal of Biological Chemistry International J. of Biological Chemistry* 1, no. 1 (2007): 69-74. doi:10.3923/ijbc.2007.69.74.

Pascual-Leone, Alvaro, Amir Amedi, Felipe Fregni, and Lotfi B. Merabet. "The Plastic Human Brain Cortex." *Annu. Rev. Neurosci. Annual Review of Neuroscience* 28, no. 1 (2005): 377-401. doi:10.1146/annurev.neuro.27.070203.144216.

Prabhala, Rao H., Harinder S. Garewal, Mary J. Hicks, Richard E. Sampliner, and Ronald R. Watson. "The Effects of 13-cis-retinoic Acid and Beta-carotene on Cellular Immunity in Humans." *Cancer* 67, no. 6 (1991): 1556-560.

doi:10.1002/1097-0142(19910315)67:63.0.co;2-0.

Prasad, AS. "Zinc in Humans Health: Effect of Zinc on Immune Cells." *Molecular Medicine: Feinstein Institute for Medical Research at N. Shore Hospital, LI* 14, no. 5-6 (May/June 2008): 353-57.

Protzko, J., J. Aronson, and C. Blair. "How to Make a Young Child Smarter: Evidence from the Database of Raising Intelligence." *Perspectives on Psychological Science* 8, no. 1 (2013): 25-40. doi:10.1177/1745691612462585.

Reuter. "Spinach Consumption Shown to Decrease Ovarian, Prostate, and Cancer Risk." *Natural Society News Letter,* June 19, 2013.

Rigacci, Stefania, Valentina Guidotti, Monica Bucciantini, Daniela Nichino, Annalisa Relini, Andrea Berti, and Massimo Stefani. "Aβ (1-42) Aggregates into Non-Toxic Amyloid Assemblies in the Presence of the Natural Polyphenol Oleuropein Aglycon." *CAR Current Alzheimer's Research* 8, no. 8 (2011): 841-52. doi:10.2174/156720511798192682.

Rudman, Daniel, Axel G. Feller, Hoskote S. Nagraj, Gregory A. Gergans, Pardee Y. Lalitha, Allen F. Goldberg, Robert A. Schlenker, Lester Cohn, Inge W. Rudman, and Dale E. Mattson. "Effects of Human Growth Hormone in Men over Sixty Years Old." *New England Journal of Medicine N Engl J Med* 323, no. 1 (1990): 1-6. doi:10.1056/nejm199007053230101.

Sacks, Frank M., George A. Bray, Vincent J. Carey, Steven R. Smith, Donna H. Ryan, Stephen D. Anton, Katherine MacManus, Catherine M. Champagne, Louise M. Bishop, Nancy Laranjo, Meryl S. Leboff, Jennifer C. Rood, Lilian De Jonge, Frank L. Greenway, Catherine M. Loria, Eva Obarzanek, and Donald A. Williamson. "Comparison of Weight-Loss Diets with Different Compositions of Fat, Protein, and Carbohydrates." *New England Journal of Medicine N Engl J Med* 360, no. 9 (2009): 859-73. doi:10.1056/nejmoa0804748.

Santos, M. S. "Beta Carotene Induced Enhancement of Natural Killer Cell Activity in Elderly Men: An Investigation of the Roles of Cytokines." *American Journal of Clinical Nutrition* 68, no. 1 (July 1998): 164-70.

Savini, Isabella, Rosaria Arnone, Maria Valeria Catani, and Luciana Avigliano. "Origanum Vulgare Induces Apoptosis in Human Colon Cancer Caco 2 Cells." *Nutrition and Cancer* 61, no. 3 (2009): 381-89. doi:10.1080/01635580802582769.

Scott, G. "Vitamin K3 (menadione) Induced Oncosis Associated with Keratin 8 Phosphorylation and Histone H3 Arylation." *Molecular Pharmacology*, 2005. doi:10.1124/mol.105.013474.

Serhan, Charles N., and Nan Chiang. "Novel Endogenous Small Molecules as the Checkpoint Controllers in Inflammation and Resolution: Entrée for Resoleomics." *Rheumatic Disease*

Clinics of North America 30, no. 1 (2004): 69-95. doi:10.1016/s0889-857x(03)00117-0.

Shah, Sachin A., Stephen Sander, C. Michael White, Mike Rinaldi, and Craig I. Coleman. "Evaluation of Echinacea for the Prevention and Treatment of the Common Cold: A Meta-analysis." *The Lancet Infectious Diseases* 7, no. 7 (2007): 473-80. doi:10.1016/s1473-3099(07)70160-3.

Shen, Chwan-Li, Kee-Jong Hong, and Sung Woo Kim. "Comparative Effects of Ginger Root (Zingiber Officinale Rosc.) on the Production of Inflammatory Mediators in Normal and Osteoarthrotic Sow Chondrocytes." *Journal of Medicinal Food* 8, no. 2 (2005): 149-53. doi:10.1089/jmf.2005.8.149.

Shug, A., D. Paulson, R. Subramanian, and V. Regitz. "Protective Effects of Propionyl-L-carnitine during Ischemia and Reperfusion." *Cardiovasc Drug Ther Cardiovascular Drugs and Therapy* 5, no. 1 (1991): 77-83. doi:10.1007/bf00128246.

Sparks, Dana. "Nutritional Supplement Can Selectively Kill Pancreatic Cancer Cells in Mice." *Mayo Clinic News Letter*, April 2, 2012.
Stefan, N., K. Kantartzis, N. Celebi, H. Staiger, J. Machann, F. Schick, A. Cegan, M. Elcnerova, E. Schleicher, A. Fritsche, and H.-U. Haring. "Circulating Palmitoleate Strongly and Independently Predicts Insulin Sensitivity in Humans." *Diabetes Care* 33, no. 2 (2009): 405-07. doi:10.2337/dc09-0544.

Szatmári, Szabolcs, and Peter Whitehouse. "Vinpocetine for Cognitive Impairment and Dementia." *Cochrane Database of Systematic Reviews* Reviews, 2003. doi:10.1002/14651858.cd003119.

Szilágyi, Géza, Zoltán Nagy, László Balkay, István Boros, Miklós Emri, Szabolcs Lehel, Teréz Márián, Tamás Molnár, Szabolcs Szakáll, Lajos Trón, Dániel Bereczki, László Csiba, István Fekete, Levente Kerényi, László Galuska, József Varga, Péter Bönöczk, Ádám Vas, and Balázs Gulyás. "Effects of Vinpocetine on the Redistribution of Cerebral Blood Flow and Glucose Metabolism in Chronic Ischemic Stroke Patients: A PET Study." *Journal of the Neurological Sciences* 229-230 (2005): 275-84. doi:10.1016/j.jns.2004.11.053.

Taglialatela, G., L. Angelucci, M.t. Ramacci, K. Werrbach-Perez, G.R. Jackson, and J.R. Perez-Polo. "Acetyl-L-Carnitine Enhances the Response of PC12 Cells to Nerve Growth Factor." *Developmental Brain Research* 59, no. 2 (1991): 221-30. doi:10.1016/0165-3806(91)90102-o.

Taglialatela, Giulio, Luciano Angelucci, Maria Teresa Ramacci, Karin Werrbach-Perez, George R. Jackson, and J. Regino Perez-Polo. "Stimulation of Nerve Growth Factor Receptors in PC12 by Acetyl-L-Carnitine." *Biochemical Pharmacology* 44, no. 3 (1992): 577-85. doi:10.1016/0006-2952(92)90452-o.

Tang, Li-Li, Rui Wang, and Xi-Can Tang. "Effects of Huperzine A on Secretion of Nerve Growth Factor in Cultured Rat Cortical Astrocytes and Neurite Outgrowth in Rat PC12 Cells." *Acta Pharmacologica Sinica* 26, no. 6 (2005): 673-78. doi:10.1111/j.1745-7254.2005.00130.x.

Tsai, Chung-Fen, Chuen-Lin Huang, Yun-Lian Lin, Yi-Chao Lee, Ying-Chen Yang, and Nai-Kuei Huang. "The Neuroprotective Effects of an Extract of Gastrodia Elata." *Journal of Ethnopharmacology* 138, no. 1 (2011): 119-25. doi:10.1016/j.jep.2011.08.064.

Victorrajmohan, Chandrasekaran, Kannampalli Pradeep, and Sivanesan Karthikeyan. "Influence of Silymarin Administration on Hepatic Glutathione-Conjugating Enzyme System in Rats Treated with Antitubercular Drugs." *Drugs in R & D* 6, no. 6 (2005): 395-400. doi:10.2165/00126839-200506060-00007.

"Vitamin D Deficiency." *New England Journal of Medicine N Engl J Med* 357, no. 19 (2007): 1980-982. doi:10.1056/nejmc072359.
Vollenhoven, Van. "Treatment of Systemic Lupus Erythematosus with DHEA." *Rheumatology* 25, no. 2 (1998): 285-89.

Vuong, T., A. Benhaddou-Andaloussi, A. Brault, D. Harbilas, L. C. Martineau, D. Vallerand, C. Ramassamy, C. Matar, and P. S. Haddad. "Anti-obesity and Anti-diabetic Effects of Bio transformed Blueberry Juice in KKAy Mice." *Int J Obes Relat Metab Disord*

International Journal of Obesity 33, no. 10 (2009): 1166-173. doi:10.1038/ijo.2009.149.

Wang, Yi Na, Yu Zhang, Yan Wang, Ding Xian Zhu, Li Qin Xu, Hong Fang, and Wei Wu. "The Beneficial Effect of Total Glucosides of Paeony on Psoriatic Arthritis Links to Circulating Tregs and Th1 Cell Function." *Phytother. Res. Phytotherapy Research* 28, no. 3 (2013): 372-81. doi:10.1002/ptr.5005.

Watkins, Bruce, Kevin Hannon, Mark Seifert, and Yong Li. "Omega-3 Fatty Acids and Bone Metabolism." *Diet, Nutrients, and Bone Health*, 2011. doi:10.1201/b11228-19.

Whitsett, T. "Resveratrol but Not EGCG, in the Diet Suppresses DMBA Mammary Cancer in Rats." *Journal of Carcinogenesis* 5, no. 15 (May 15, 2006).

Wicha, Max. "Breast Cancer Stem Cells and Response to Sulphoraphane." *University of Michigan Position Paper*, 2003.

Wong, Carmen P., Linda P. Nguyen, Sang K. Noh, Tammy M. Bray, Richard S. Bruno, and Emily Ho. "Induction of Regulatory T Cells by Green Tea Polyphenol EGCG." *Immunology Letters* 139, no. 1-2 (2011): 7-13. doi:10.1016/j.imlet.2011.04.009.

Wong, George Y.C., Leon Bradlow, Daniel Sepkovic, Stephanie Mehl, Joshua Mailman, and Michael P. Osborne. "Dose-ranging Study of Indole-3-Carbinol for Breast Cancer

Prevention." *Journal of Cellular Biochemistry J. Cell. Biochem.* 67, no. S28-29 (1997): 111-16. doi:10.1002/(sici)1097-4644(1997)28/29 3.0.co;2-k.

Yang, Zhi-Hong, Hiroko Miyahara, and Akimasa Hatanaka. "Chronic Administration of Palmitoleic Acid Reduces Insulin Resistance and Hepatic Lipid Accumulation in KK-Ay Mice with Genetic Type 2 Diabetes." *Lipids Health Dis Lipids in Health and Disease* 10, no. 1 (2011): 120. doi:10.1186/1476-511x-10-120.

Yegenoglu, Hande, Belma Aslim, and Feyza Oke. "Comparison of Antioxidant Capacities of Ganoderma Lucidum (Curtis) P. Karst and Funalia Trogii (Berk.) Bondartsev & Singer by Using Different In Vitro Methods." *Journal of Medicinal Food* 14, no. 5 (2011): 512-16. doi:10.1089/jmf.2010.0144.

Yeung, Fan, Jamie E. Hoberg, Catherine S. Ramsey, Michael D. Keller, David R. Jones, Roy A. Frye, and Marty W. Mayo. "Modulation of NF-κB-dependent Transcription and Cell Survival by the SIRT1 Deacetylase." *EMBO J The EMBO Journal* 23, no. 12 (2004): 2369-380. doi:10.1038/sj.emboj.7600244.

Yu, Weiping, Sook-Kyung Park, Li Jia, Richa Tiwary, Wenjun W. Scott, Jing Li, Pei Wang, Marla Simmons-Menchaca, Bob G. Sanders, and Kimberly Kline. "RRR-γ-tocopherol Induces Human Breast Cancer Cells to Undergo Apoptosis via Death Receptor 5 (DR5)-mediated Apoptotic Signaling." *Cancer Letters* 259, no. 2 (2008): 165-76.

doi:10.1016/j.canlet.2007.10.008.

Yuan, Jian-Min. "Green Tea and Prevention of Esophageal and Lung Cancers." *Molecular Nutrition & Food Research Mol. Nutr. Food Res.* 55, no. 6 (2011): 886-904. doi:10.1002/mnfr.201000637.

Zhang, Ke, Xu Ma, Wenjun He, Haixia Li, Shuyan Han, Yong Jiang, Hounan Wu, Li Han, Tomohiro Ohno, Nobuo Uotsu, Kohji Yamaguchi, Zhizhong Ma, and Pengfei Tu. "Extracts of Cistanche Deserticola Can Antagonize Immunosenescense and Extend Life Span in Senescence-Accelerated Mouse Prone 8 (SAM-P8) Mice." *Evidence-Based Complementary and Alternative Medicine* 2014 (2014): 1-14. doi:10.1155/2014/601383.

Zhang, Lian, Junling Ma, Kaifeng Pan, Vay Liang W. Go, Junshi Chen, and Wei-Cheng You. "Efficacy of Cranberry Juice on Helicobacter Pylori Infection: A Double-Blind, Randomized Placebo-Controlled Trial." *Helicobacter* 10, no. 2 (2005): 139-45. doi:10.1111/j.1523-5378.2005.00301.x.

Zhang, Yan-Jie, Yanwen Duan, and X.F. Steven Zheng. "Targeting the MTOR Kinase Domain: The Second Generation of MTOR Inhibitors." *Drug Discovery Today* 16, no. 7-8 (2011): 325-31. doi:10.1016/j.drudis.2011.02.008.

Zhang, Zhao, Pu Ma, Younian Xu, Meijun Zhan, Yunjian Zhang, Shanglong Yao, and Shihai Zhang. "Preventive Effect of Gastrodin on Cognitive Decline after Cardiac Surgery with Cardiopulmonary Bypass: A Double-blind, Randomized Controlled Study." *Journal of Huazhong University of Science and Technology [Medical Sciences] J. Huazhong Univ. Sci. Technol. [Med. Sci.]* 31, no. 1 (2011): 120-27. doi:10.1007/s11596-011-0162-4.

ABOUT THE AUTHOR

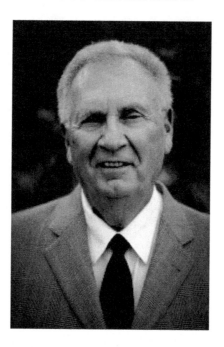

Dr. David L. Vastola is Board Certified in Internal Medicine and Gastroenterologist who has done extensive clinical research proving that taking vitamins, minerals, and herbal supplements are a sensible precaution to avoiding nutrient deficiencies common throughout life. He believes specific nutrient replacement and positive communication between the patient and physician, as well as being diligent and proactive, are the keys to staying healthy and avoiding the aging process. He runs a private practice in Palm Beach Gardens, Florida, specializing in Internal Medicine and Gastroenterology, and is often called the "Sherlock Holmes of Medicine" for uncovering problems other medical professionals missed.

He has written four books, been married for thirty-five years, has five children, employs an assistant lovingly named Patrick the Poodle, and is showcasing a new TV pilot called *Good Health Hunting* at four film festivals.

Dr. Vastola has extensive media experience as a medical and nutrition expert on WJNO Radio for twenty years in southeast Florida, local TV Fox News five days a week for eight years, as well as CBS local News. Nationally, he has been on CNN and was quoted in *The Wall Street Journal*. http://www.yourgoodhealthfl.com/

Made in the USA
Middletown, DE
15 January 2021

31647240R00136